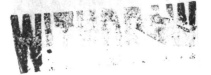

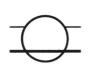

FEMALE FORMS

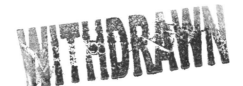

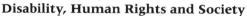

Disability, Human Rights and Society

Series Editor: Professor Len Barton, University of Sheffield

The *Disability, Human Rights and Society* series reflects a commitment to a particular view of 'disability' and a desire to make this view accessible to a wider audience. The series approach defines 'disability' as a form of oppression and identifies the ways in which disabled people are marginalized, restricted and experience discrimination. The fundamental issue is not one of an individual's inabilities or limitations, but rather a hostile and unadaptive society.

Authors in this series are united in the belief that the question of disability must be set within an equal opportunities framework. The series gives priority to the examination and critique of those factors that are unacceptable, offensive and in need of change. It also recognizes that any attempt to redirect resources in order to provide opportunities for discriminated people cannot pretend to be apolitical. Finally, it raises the urgent task of establishing links with other marginalized groups in an attempt to engage in a common struggle. The issue of disability needs to be given equal significance to those of race, gender and age in equal opportunities policies. This series provides support for such a task.

Anyone interested in contributing to the series is invited to approach the Series Editor at the Department of Educational Studies, University of Sheffield.

Current and forthcoming titles

F. Armstrong and L. Barton: *Disability, Human Rights and Education: Cross-Cultural Perspectives*

M. Corker: *Deaf and Disabled, or Deafness Disabled?: Towards a Human Rights Perspective*

M. Corker and S. French (eds): *Disability Discourse*

M. Moore, S. Beazley and J. Maelzer: *Researching Disability Issues*

J. Read: *The Mediators: Mothers of Disabled Children and the Social Order*

A. Roulstone: *Enabling Technology: Disabled People, Work and New Technology*

C. Thomas: *Female Forms: Experiencing and Understanding Disability*

A. Vlachou: *Struggles for Inclusive Education: An Ethnographic Study*

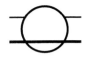

FEMALE FORMS
Experiencing and understanding disability

Carol Thomas

Open University Press
Buckingham · Philadelphia

Open University Press
Celtic Court
22 Ballmoor
Buckingham
MK18 1XW

e-mail: enquiries@openup.co.uk
world wide web: http://www.openup.co.uk

and
325 Chestnut Street
Philadelphia, PA 19106, USA

First Published 1999

A catalogue record of this book is available from the British Library

ISBN   0 335 19693 4 (pb)   0 335 19694 2 (hb)

Library of Congress Cataloging-in-Publication Data
Thomas, Carol, 1958–
    Female Forms : experiencing and understanding disability / Carol Thomas.
      p.   cm. – (Disability, human rights, and society)
    Includes bibliographical references.
    ISBN 0-335-19694-2. – ISBN 0-335-19693-4 (pbk.)
    1. Disability studies–Great Britain.   2. Handicapped women–Great Britain.
3. Feminist theory–Great Britain.   I. Title. II. Series.
HV1568.25.G7T46   1999
362.4'082'0941–dc21   98-55530
                                                    CIP

Typeset by Type Study, Scarborough

Printed and bound in Great Britain by
Marston Lindsay Ross International Ltd,
Oxfordshire

To the memory of my mother, Moyra Thomas

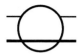

Contents

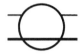

Series editor's preface

The Disability, Human Rights and Society Series reflects a commitment to a social model of disability and a desire to make this view accessible to a wide audience. 'Disability' is viewed as a form of oppression and the fundamental issue is not one of an individual's inabilities or limitations, but rather a hostile and unadaptive society.

Priority is given to identifying and challenging those barriers to change, including the urgent task of establishing links with other marginalized groups and thus seeking to make connections between class, gender, race, age and disability factors.

The series aims to further establish disability as a serious topic of study, one in which the latest research findings and ideas can be seriously engaged with.

Disability Studies within higher education in Britain in particular, has been characterized by a commitment to a social model of disability. This approach has been significantly influenced by historical materialist and feminist ideas and concerns. In this book Thomas reinforces a recognition of such contributions and by critically engaging with existing ideas, offers a series of perspectives that are intended to move forward ways of defining, understanding and explaining disability and impairment.

A key theoretical question reflecting the author's personal perspective and which the reader needs to be aware of is, 'how are the social relationships which constitute disability generated and sustained within social and cultural formations?' (p. 2). This interest provides Thomas with the motivation to consider several key themes including: the gendered nature of disability; the nature of social oppression, taking the experiential seriously; difference and identity. A particular interest is that of encouraging a constructive dialogue between disability studies and medical sociology.

One of the great strengths of the book is the ways in which Thomas has carefully used the powerful narratives of a group of disabled women. Much of this material is highly informative, and powerfully illustrates their perspectives and experiences. They are thoughtful and thought-provoking accounts and provide a wealth of rich insights for reflection and discussion. Thomas acknowledges how these insider perspectives had a formative influence on her thinking and the development of this book. As a reader I found them to be challenging and stimulating, causing me to reconsider existing understandings and to confront alternative perspectives.

This book has been written in a most lucid, informative and accessible style. A contributory factor has been the way in which the author's interest in the experiential, has resulted in sensitive and skilful ways of writing herself into the text. This has provided an additional means of sustaining the reader's interest.

I do hope that this book receives a wide readership as I have no doubt that it will provoke discussion and stimulate an informed re-examination of many key ideas and understandings currently available. This includes both theoretical and socio-practical implementations.

The book is essential reading for all those interested in issues of social exclusion and inclusion and will make an important contribution to the development of Disability Studies.

Professor Len Barton
Sheffield

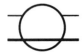

Acknowledgements

There are many people who have influenced my thinking about disability, and have contributed to the making of this book in one way or another. I am grateful to the Leverhulme Trust for the award of a research fellowship without which the book would not have been written. Special thanks go to all the women who communicated with me about their experiences. The following colleagues and friends are owed thanks for supporting me in their different ways – meeting with me, commenting on my work in this field, sharing literature and ideas, being patient with me as other work took second place: Alison Hayward, Jenny Morris, Mike Oliver, Janet Price, Mairian Corker, Hilary Graham, Jackie Stacey, Bev Skeggs, Gareth Williams, Heather Wilkinson, Lisa Bostock, Sara Morris, Tony Gatrell, Penny Curtis, Karen Dunn, Jan Rigby and Pat Clelland. I am grateful to Jennie Popay and David Clark for supporting my Leverhulme application, and to David Smith and other colleagues in the Department of Applied Social Science at Lancaster University. I also owe much to those involved in the Institute for Women's Studies at Lancaster University, some already mentioned. Thanks to Jacinta Evans at Open University Press, and to Len Barton for his helpful comments. Particular thanks go, as ever, to Quentin Rudland and Jay Rudland-Thomas.

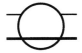

Introduction

Understanding disability

What is disability? How can it be explained and theorized? Increasingly, disabled people have come to reject commonplace ideas which suggest either that disability *is* an impairment, chronic illness, or medical condition ('my disability is that I cannot walk', 'her disability is that she has epilepsy'), or that disability is the restricted activity caused by impairment ('because she cannot walk she is disabled in everyday life'). The disabled people's movement in Britain and internationally, together with writers and researchers in Disability Studies, have developed their own understanding of disability. In Britain, this relatively new way of thinking about disability is known as the *social model of disability*. Social modellists break the old links between disability and impairment, so that disability is seen not as the impairment itself, nor as being caused by impairment. Disability is redefined as the outcome of social arrangements and practices which work to exclude and disadvantage people with impairment; social barriers place restrictions on what they can do and how they can live. In this way, disability becomes a new form of social oppression.

This book is a critical engagement with the ideas about disability and impairment which have emerged within Disability Studies in the last two decades, focusing principally but not exclusively on published work in Britain. It attempts to convey the wealth of ideas which have been unleashed by the social modellist reformulation of disability (both in its favour and against it), and to contribute to the further development of the social theorization of disability. It also considers differences in approach to the study of disability between Disability Studies and medical sociology.

The title, *Female Forms*, reflects two important themes. The first is my particular interest in the lives of disabled women, being one myself. I was born without a left hand, and I have a personal commitment to Disability Studies and disability politics. As a sociologist with a long-standing interest in women's studies, I wanted to write a book which drew on the experiences of disabled women, including my own, but which was also of general relevance. The challenge was to use women's experiences to illustrate the gendered nature of disability whilst at the same time developing ideas about disability which are of significance for all. The second feature is the book's engagement with, and use of, feminist perspectives. Disability Studies, I suggest, can learn a great deal of value from the work of feminist authors, and the book pays particular attention to what disabled feminists have had to say on the subject of disability and impairment.

The book is not simply 'feminist', however. It develops a materialist feminist understanding of disability, drawing on historical materialist premises and feminist scholarship, where I see these as compatible. I have disagreements with both the type of materialist analyses which are associated with the work of influential social modellists in Britain, most notably Mike Oliver (1990; 1992; 1996a; 1996b; 1996c; 1997), and with postmodernist and poststructuralist perspectives in Disability Studies as well as in feminism more generally. Much of the discussion in this book is concerned with outlining, as well as critiquing, the contrasting ways in which disability and impairment can be understood when different theoretical perspectives within the social sciences are employed.

I have written this text with different audiences in mind. The book has something to say to students, academics and researchers in a number of fields, especially Disability Studies, women's studies, medical sociology, and the health and social care professions. I hope that it will also be of interest to activists and lay readers in the disabled people's movement and beyond. To serve these readerships, I have attempted to give accessible accounts of a wide range of ideas and debates about disability, to reference carefully, and to present my own analysis in a stepwise fashion. With each successive chapter new elements of my argument about disability and impairment are built in. Thus my analysis unfolds and develops in a linear fashion, and can best be appreciated by reading the chapters in order.

The structure of the book and the argument

The book is organized into three parts. Part I, 'Defining Disability', consists of three chapters which explore, from different angles, what disability is and what it encompasses. The discussion in each chapter assists in the clarification of what I see as the key theoretical question: how are the social relationships which constitute disability generated and sustained within social and cultural formations?

Chapter 1 traces the development of the social model of disability and the emergence of Disability Studies. The gendered nature of disability is introduced, as are a growing number of critiques of the social model from within Disability Studies itself. The strength and importance of the social model perspective as a starting point is underlined, using disabled women's narratives as illustrative (the source of these narratives is discussed below).

The purpose of Chapter 2 is to outline and resolve what I have called a definitional riddle about disability. To explain this riddle, an authoritative definitional schema which is rejected by social modellists is discussed: the *International Classification of Impairments, Disabilities and Handicaps* (ICIDH) (Wood 1980). The work of two authors who use this schema, one a British-based medical sociologist and the other a Canadian-based feminist author, is discussed. This sets the scene for examining what I call the *social relational* and the *property* approaches to defining disability, both of which are found in the work of social modellists in Disability Studies. I advance the argument that the frequent conflation of the social relational and property definitions of disability is confusing and unhelpful. I suggest that what is needed in Disability Studies is the consistent usage of a social relational understanding of disability. Chapter 2 also discusses the importance of acknowledging and understanding what I call *impairment effects*.

Chapter 3 makes a case for extending a social relational understanding of disability so that it encompasses not only social processes and practices which prevent people with impairment from 'doing' things (for example, getting paid employment, succeeding in education, accessing suitable housing), but also those disablist social processes and practices which damage our quality of 'being', that is, which undermine what I refer to as our *psycho-emotional well-being*. Once again, disabled women's own accounts of living with disability are drawn upon to illustrate the argument. Chapter 3 also reviews some of the work within Disability Studies which emphasizes the importance of cultural processes in explaining disability, and the ensuing debate about whether the social model can accommodate cultural matters. By the end of Part I, I can offer my preferred definition of disability: *disability is a form of social oppression involving the social imposition of restrictions of activity on people with impairments and the socially engendered undermining of their psycho-emotional well-being.*

Part II, 'Female Forms', consists of three chapters which consider the importance of feminist perspectives for Disability Studies. Chapter 4 discusses the place of 'personal experience' in Disability Studies. Feminists have long argued that 'the personal is political', and disabled feminist writers such as Jenny Morris (1991; 1992a; 1993a; 1993b; 1995; 1996) have brought this perspective into their disability research. This has engendered a hostile reaction in some quarters in Disability Studies, most clearly expressed in Vic Finkelstein's (1996: 34) statement that focusing on personal experience is a 'discredited and sterile approach to understanding and changing the world'. Mike Oliver (1996a; 1996b) has also argued against calls by Liz Crow (1996) and Jenny Morris (1996) for account to be taken of personal experiences of living with impairment. This debate about personal experience (of disability, impairment, or both) is considered in the light of feminist analyses of epistemology (theories of knowledge) in the social sciences. I argue, in line with feminist perspectives more generally, that there are very sound reasons for taking the experiential seriously, including: 'writing the self' into one's analysis, reflexivity, and the utilization of what sociologists have termed 'auto/biography'. I demonstrate that old and unsustainable dualisms which separate the personal from the political, the private from the social, are found lurking not far beneath the arguments used by Oliver, Finkelstein and others against engaging with personal experience.

In Chapter 5, the gendered nature of disability is discussed in some detail. This chapter draws heavily on disabled women's personal accounts of their day-to-day lives. The women's narratives illustrate that the forms and impacts of disablism are invariably refracted in some way through the prism of gender locations and gender relations. The narratives also tell of how disabled women continuously exercise their agency in resisting and transgressing oppressive boundaries. The chapter closes with a discussion of the difficulties in theorizing the gender–disability interface.

This leads into a detailed consideration of 'difference' in Chapter 6. Theorizing difference has become an important undertaking within feminism, particularly differences associated with gender, 'race'[1] and sexuality. Feminist debate on theorizing difference is briefly outlined, especially the distinction between essentialist and constructionist approaches. Attention then turns to the contrasting ways in which a number of disabled feminist authors, namely Susan Wendell, Jenny Morris, Janet Price (and her co-writers), and Mairian Corker, have dealt with difference – especially differences between disabled and non-disabled people. Chapter 6 also touches on the question of 'identity' and identity politics. The chapter closes with some reflections on debates about difference and identity. I explain my view that the essentialist versus constructionist paradigm is of limited usefulness because it elides explanatory approaches which seek to be materialist, or realist, *but not* biologically or socially reductionist.

Part III, 'Understanding Disability', consists of two chapters, and delves more deeply into theoretical approaches. Chapter 7 begins with a summary of the conceptual threads in my own analysis of disability and impairment, then outlines two broad theoretical paradigms which are particularly influential in Disability Studies at present: historical materialism and postmodernism. The underlying premises of these perspectives are considered, together with a review of their applications in Disability Studies. The final section reiterates my own leanings towards materialist feminist perspectives, and considers ways forward for theoretical work on disability and impairment.

Chapter 8 examines the 'divide' between Disability Studies and medical sociology, focusing on three areas: the conceptualization of disability, understanding experience, and the practice of disability research. This chapter is included because an exploration of the different approaches used in Disability Studies and medical sociology can assist in clarifying ideas about disability. I have learned a great deal from medical sociology as well as from Disability Studies, and, whilst recognizing the problems, would like to encourage further dialogue between the two.

Experiencing disability: disabled women's narratives

A number of chapters include women's personal accounts of their experiences of living with disability. I have introduced these narratives, sometimes at length, to bring the themes in this book to life, and because they are richly informative in their own right. They inject a 'down to earth' quality into what would otherwise be a very abstract discussion of ideas and concepts. In my view, these personal accounts are singular in their power to illustrate and illuminate. I now want to explain how I came by this narrative material, which I have also used in work on growing up with disability (Thomas 1998b), narrative identity (Thomas 1999), and disabled women becoming mothers (Thomas 1997, 1998a). In presenting narratives, I have endeavoured to protect identities by changing names, and omitting place names and other identifying details.[2]

In January 1996 I sent out a 'press release' to over 150 disability organizations (mainly national ones) listed in the 1995–96 *Disability Rights Handbook* (Disability Alliance Educational and Research Association 1995). The press release told women that I was undertaking research for a book on women and disability, that I was a disabled woman myself, that I was looking for first-hand accounts of living with disability so that 'women's voices' could be represented in my work. It listed 14 areas of social and personal life which were of interest. Women were invited to write to me, send a self-recorded tape, or communicate in some other way. I had no control over how the press release was used by the organizations it was sent to, but in the main it seems to have been reproduced, in part or as a whole, in newsletters to members.

The press release generated a surprisingly large response over a period of 12 months. I received over 80 telephone calls, letters, e-mails and faxes from all over the UK. These first contacts were usually to find out more about what I was doing and to clarify what I wanted. Then came the more substantial letters, other written 'articles' and pieces of varying lengths and levels of detail, including some comprehensive 'life story' papers, and some self-recorded tapes. Written material was received from 49 women, and self-recorded tapes from five more. The written material included a book which one correspondent had published about her life experiences; she generously sent me a copy (Berwick 1990). Where women lived within a reasonable distance from Lancaster University, I arranged to interview them in their homes, or at the University if they preferred. Two of these interviews were with women who lived further afield, but they were so keen to meet that they elected to travel considerable distances to the University. Fourteen interviews were conducted; thus, in total, I obtained accounts from 68 women.

In many cases a dialogue was entered into; typically a first contact was made with me by telephone or in writing, a discussion then took place about my research, and then I was sent a letter or self-recorded tape. I sometimes wrote back asking for further information on particular points, and a second letter would follow. Two years on, I still enjoy communication with a few of the women. A snowball process was set in motion – some women suggested that a disabled friend might be interested in telling me of their experiences. A few of the interviews and letters came about in this way. Thus I found myself in a 'dialogic' research process such that the end 'data products' were, in most instances, generated through an interaction with individuals through various media over time. This often meant sharing some of my own experiences, thoughts and feelings with the women. However, I endeavoured to ensure that the women who communicated their stories were very much in control of what they disclosed. This was particularly true of the majority who sent in written pieces or self-recorded tapes, but is inevitably less true of the interviews where I played a more significant role in shaping the discourse. Despite the fact that most of those who wrote to me had seen the full press release with its list of areas of interest, had talked with me on the telephone, and/or had received a letter from me asking for more information on particular points, I would argue that they could dictate the content and form of the material they gave me to a greater extent than most respondents are able to in social research. This, I would suggest, is a strength rather than a weakness of the research. The listing of areas of interest in the press release was broad enough to signal that I was interested in all and any aspects of social life and personal experience.[3] Some women chose to use the list as an organizing framework – moving through the headings in turn in their letters or tapes. Others communicated on only one, two or a few specific areas. The items listed in the press release did not play a prescriptive but a facilitating role, and I am certain that by naming areas such as 'sex, sexuality, sexual relationships' and 'abuse – physical, emotional, sexual' the women were 'given permission' to communicate about very painful personal experiences, on which they might otherwise have remained silent.

This method of gathering information about disability experiences inevitably resulted in non-standardized material of a very disparate character, and the 'respondents' were self-selected. Many of the women told me that they were motivated to participate by their belief – a well-founded one, I hope – that by making their voices heard they were doing something that would contribute towards improving the lot of disabled women in our society. Of course, the 'sample' of participating women cannot be claimed to be representative of disabled women in a statistical sense. However, it is important to note that ages were fairly evenly distributed through the twenties, thirties, forties and fifties, with some in the sixties and seventies. A wide range of physical and sensory impairments were represented. Some women had multiple impairments, some had lived with impairment since birth, whilst others had acquired or developed impairment(s) in childhood or adulthood. Included were women who were relatively recently impaired, women living with chronic illness and deteriorating health, and some whose physical or sensory state was relatively stable. However, one group of women who were very under-represented are those with learning difficulty. I now regret that I did not make more of an effort to reach these women, and find ways of enabling them to share their experiences with me. Other women whose narratives are notably absent are disabled black and minority ethnic women. I appear to have failed to reach and engage the interest of such women, and the absence of their stories is a major omission (the press release was purposively sent to self-declared black disability organizations). Thankfully, sexualities were not exclusively heterosexual, and personal circumstances and geographical locations differed markedly. Socio-economic, educational and familial experiences were very variable.

Thus, despite its shortcomings, the 'sample' of women who entered into dialogue with me constituted a variable, yet at the same time 'ordinary', cross-section of disabled women. With a few exceptions, it was clear from their accounts that these were not political activists in the disabled people's movement, and most would not have considered themselves feminists. In the main, they were not women who were used to publicly expressing their views, although many were members of disability organizations (usually impairment-specific national organizations) and some did paid or voluntary work for local disability organizations and groups.

It is important to understand that these women's narratives, like any other personal accounts, do not give us direct, or unmediated, access to life experiences (related epistemological matters are discussed in Chapter 4). Narratives are representations, involving interpretation and selection in their construction (the 'telling'), in their consumption (my 'reading'), in their reproduction (my 're-presentation'), and in their further interpretation (your 'reading') (Riessman 1993). As the author of this book, and like any other researcher, I have inevitably selected narratives which best support *my own* interpretation and analysis of the issue in question (having given due attention to all the evidence). In fact, it took me some time to decide how precisely to use and present the information which women imparted in the ways described. It was never my intention to write a book which was simply an analysis of these data. Rather, my plan was to use the material for illustrative purposes, treating it as a source of examples and quotations. However, influenced by seminar events and literature on the use of both auto/biography and narrative analysis (in feminism and sociology),[4] I eventually opted to maintain the integrity and storied quality of the narratives by reproducing, largely unedited, quite lengthy sections from the letters, self-recorded tapes and interview transcripts. This has inevitably placed a limit on the number of women whose accounts could be included, and selection within accounts was still required.

Nevertheless, all of the narrative material had a formative impact on my thinking in one way or another, and thus played a role in shaping the content of this book. I found many of the things that the women told me surprising and novel, and my preconceptions were often challenged. Their narratives offered insights which broadened my perspective and frequently forced me to rethink. Apart from anything else, the narratives demonstrated that, from the perspective of lived experience, the effects of living with both *disability* and what I have called *impairment effects* are closely intermeshed, and together shape what we do and who we are.

Key terms

The book devotes a considerable amount of space to discussing what I and others mean by the term 'disability', so I will not dwell on it here. It is necessary, however, to say something about the meaning I give to the follow-ing frequently used terms: Disability Studies, social oppression and impair-ment.

The term 'Disability Studies' is used to refer to those academics, writers and researchers who, in studying disability, explicitly align themselves with the social movement for the advancement of the social and political rights of dis-abled people. Many, but not all, of those involved in Disability Studies are themselves disabled, and many are also activists in the disabled people's movement. In the UK, the hallmark of belonging to Disability Studies is some kind of adherence to the social model of disability (even as a prelude to heav-ily critiquing it).

The term 'social oppression' is quite difficult to define. It is widely used in analyses of the social position of groups who, in material and intangible ways, are systematically disadvantaged *vis-à-vis* others: women *vis-à-vis* men; black people *vis-à-vis* white people; gays and lesbians *vis-à-vis* straight people, the old *vis-à-vis* the young; working-class people *vis-à-vis* members of the affluent classes. Issues of power imbalance, the systematization of privilege and under-privilege, the structural reproduction of inequality, the institutionalization of disadvantage, are all at stake here. This book follows others in adding disabled people to the list of those who are socially oppressed, or, to use a more recent term, *socially excluded*. The challenge is to understand the nature and reasons for this form of social oppression.

Of course, unlike some other oppressed sections of society, disabled people include among their number many who have moved from the ranks of the non-disabled (the non-oppressed, at least in this connection) into the com-pany of 'the disabled' (the oppressed) – as they acquire impairments, most commonly with advancing age. Disability Studies has shown that this difficult transition is not just about learning to live with the immediate effects of trauma or long-term illness (important though this is), but is fundamentally about discovering the myriad ways in which lives now come to be shaped and limited by disablism. Social oppressions intersect in ways which we are only beginning to explore.

In this book, the term 'impairment' (and its derivatives: physical, sensory and intellectual impairment) is not treated as a taken-for-granted, or unprob-lematized, referent to 'abnormal' features of the body or the biological. Nor do I see human bodies simply as biological entities which exist in some kind of independent, fixed, unchanging, or universalistic state.

First, the term impairment, like any other linguistic category, is a social product, and as such possesses a cultural history (belonging to particular times and places). With this in mind, 'impairments' can be understood to be those *variations* in the structure, function and workings of bodies which, in Western culture, are medically defined as significant abnormalities or pathologies. Thus, in my case, having been born with only one hand (a clear-cut variation from the usual) is socio-medically defined as a 'significant deviation from the normal type' and labels me as a 'person with impairment'. It is important to note that this qualified way of understanding 'impairment' lies behind the usage of the term in what follows (I have refrained from boring the reader by spelling it out every time). Of course, these kinds of 'significant variations' continue to be 'discovered' and catalogued by medical science through detailed diagnostic labelling and categorization,[5] most recently in the field of genetics with the Human Genome Project. This sociological starting point (that the category 'impairment' is socially produced), is taken much further by some who adopt postmodernist and poststructuralist perspectives, as will be discussed at some length in Chapters 6 and 7. From their constructionist point of view, impairment (the 'signifier') is seen to be entirely constituted through discursive practices and has no necessary relationship to any 'real' bodily state (the 'signified'); this is not a view which I share. The anthropological study of the social meanings and consequences connected with 'unusual' bodily features or attributes is beyond the scope of this book, but is of undoubted significance for Disability Studies (see, for example, Scheer and Groce 1988; Oliver 1990; Barnes 1996; 1997a; Shakespeare 1997a).

Second, in my view it is too limiting to think of impairment as connected with a biological substratum, 'the human body', which is fixed (albeit overlaid with social meanings which change in time and place). Rather, this 'biological substratum' is itself a social product, as well as a physically changing 'biological' entity. Human bodies possess a materiality which exists in a relationship of dynamic interaction with its social and physical environment. Put simply, bodies shape these environments through their (purposive) activity, and these environments shape the body – giving rise both to some bodily variations themselves, and to the meanings and significance which these variations come to have. Paul Abberley (1987; 1996; 1997) has drawn attention to the social creation of impairment, and his work is discussed in Chapter 7.

Notes

1 Following sociological convention, the term race appears in inverted commas: 'race'. This indicates that, whilst it remains a widely used term for the purpose of distinguishing between groups who vary culturally, in terms of physical characteristics, and in terms of power and privilege, there are, in fact, no biologically distinct races among humans.

2 In writing this book I was faced with the dilemma that some of my correspondents were quite happy for me to use their real names and other identifying details (indeed, some would have preferred this), whilst most wanted the assurance of confidentiality. I decided to be consistent and *always* change names and protect confidentiality as far as possible (unless dealing with material already published in the name of the author). This is because it is quite possible that correspondents might regret the revelation of their identity at a later date. I can only apologize to any correspondent I may offend by my decision.

3 The list was as follows:

- What is it like to use health and welfare services?
- Experiences of health and welfare professionals/workers.

- Care: being 'cared for', being 'independent'. Carers – family, friends or professionals/workers.
- Paid work and work in the home (housework and childcare).
- Personal relationships – with parents, family, lovers, husbands, partners, children.
- Sex, sexuality, sexual relationships.
- Abuse – physical, emotional, sexual.
- Issues to do with having or not having children.
- Living arrangements, housing.
- Money, income, benefits.
- Education.
- Feelings about yourself. Have these changed?
- Health and well-being.
- Getting involved in groups, campaigns and so on.

4 I am fortunate in being based at Lancaster University, where there is a vibrant intellectual culture, not least associated with the Institute for Women's Studies. Among other things, the Institute was involved in the organization of a seminar series, funded by the Economic and Social Research Council (ESRC), on feminism and auto/biography in 1997–98. My approach in this book has undoubtedly been influenced by what I learned as a regular participant in these excellent seminars. I have also delved into some of the literature on the sociology of auto/biography (Sociology 1993; Somers 1994), narrative analysis (Riessman 1993), feminist praxis (Stanley 1990), and the sociology of story-telling (Plummer 1995).

5 Those engaged in medical, paramedical or health services research use a wide range of terms to define and describe impairment, including: pathology, disease, injury, trauma, congenital/developmental conditions, dysfunctions, structural abnormalities in specific body systems (musculoskeletal, cardiovascular, neurological etc.), functional limitations or restrictions in basic physical and mental actions (ambulating, reaching, stooping, climbing, producing intelligible speech, seeing standard print, hearing standard sounds, etc.).

PART I

DEFINING DISABILITY

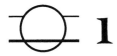 **1**

Defining disability: the social model

Introduction

When socially disadvantaged individuals and groups to whom a label such as 'disabled' has been applied begin to unsettle the status quo by demanding social justice and equality, the terms which have been unquestioningly used come to be critically scrutinized by those so labelled, and are either rejected or 'owned' but radically redefined. So it was with terms such as 'queer' or 'black', and in the last 30 years the same has occurred with the term 'disabled'. This chapter begins by outlining the way in which the disabled people's movement in Britain has redefined disability in terms of the *social model of disability*. Taking the work of the disabled activist and scholar, Mike Oliver (1990; 1996a; 1996b; 1996c), as the exemplar, I will discuss the features of the social model and consider its challenge to conventional ways of thinking about what disability is. The social model of disability has become the conceptualization of disability with most resonance and support in the British disabled people's movement, and, as such, is the reference point for those both within and outside that movement and Disability Studies who want to take a social understanding of disability further, or in different directions. Particularly in Britain, authors tend to define their positions in relation to the social model of disability.

This chapter outlines the social model and its political roots, illustrates the model's perspective by drawing on women's narratives, briefly introduces a range of criticisms of it which have emerged within Disability Studies in recent years, and begins to consider the issue of gender differences. The social model is also my own point of departure, and the discussion sets the scene for the development of my analytical perspective in subsequent chapters. Throughout this chapter and those which follow, for any definition of disability under discussion, a shorthand version of the causal relationship proposed is given in parentheses. For example, Oliver's social model definition of disability proposes that disability is caused by 'social barriers', and this is represented as (Social barriers → Disability), the arrow signalling the relationship between cause and effect. This device is used to summarize the essential (but sometimes subtle) differences between definitional approaches.

Political roots

In the last 30 years in Britain a social definition of disability has emerged from within the organizations *of* (as opposed to *for*) disabled people (Campbell and Oliver 1996). This social definition, now widely referred to as the social model of disability, was first formulated in the struggle of disability activists to carve out some 'fundamental principles' on disability as the basis of a political programme (for a summary of this, see Oliver 1996b), and it became the distinguishing feature of the conceptual framework used by a number of influential 'disability theorists' (Oliver 1990; 1996b; Swain *et al.* 1993; Barton 1996a; Campbell and Oliver 1996; Barton and Oliver 1997). There is now a rapidly growing Disability Studies literature using this perspective as its starting point.[1]

The social model asserts that it is not the individual's impairment which causes disability (Impairment → Disability), or which *is* the disability (Impairment = Disability), and it is not the difficulty of individual functioning with physical, sensory or intellectual impairment which generates the problems of disability. Rather, disability is the outcome of social arrangements which work to restrict the activities of people with impairments by placing *social barriers* in their way (Social barriers → Disability). This social causation, or social creation, of disability is sometimes referred to as the 'social construction' of disability.[2]

In Britain, the original, and now 'classic', formulation identifying disability as socially caused is found in the 'Fundamental Principles of Disability' document of the Union of the Physically Impaired Against Segregation (UPIAS), written in 1976 (reproduced in part in Oliver 1996b). This organization, formed in 1972, played a critical intellectual and political role in disability politics in Britain in the 1970s (Campbell and Oliver 1996).

UPIAS definitions of impairment and disability

Impairment: 'lacking all of part of a limb, or having a defective limb, organ or mechanism of the body'.

Disability: 'the disadvantage or restriction of activity caused by a contemporary social organisation which takes no or little account of people who have physical impairments and thus excludes them from the mainstream of social activities' (Oliver 1996b: 22)

Colin Barnes (1996), a disabled activist and scholar, has explained how this socio-political definition of disability, with its reference to physical impairments, was subsequently broadened to accommodate all impairments – physical, sensory and intellectual – by successive organizations of disabled people such as the British Council of Organisations of Disabled People (BCODP).[3] A modified version of these definitions was also adopted by the Disabled People's International (DPI).[4]

DPI definitions of impairment and disability

Impairment: 'the functional limitation within the individual caused by physical, mental or sensory impairment'.

Disability: 'the loss or limitation of opportunities to take part in the normal life of the community on an equal level with others due to physical and social barriers' (DPI 1982, cited in Oliver 1996a: 41).

The social model of disability signals a radical shift in thinking about disability, recasting disability as a form of social oppression. As Paul Abberley (1987) argued in the late 1980s, disablism joins sexism, racism, homophobia and ageism in the catalogue of social oppressions. The social model throws the spotlight on the need for societal change and the removal of socially created barriers and all forms of institutional discrimination (Barnes 1991), in contrast to the 'help the unfortunate disabled person to adjust to their limitations' perspective which has dominated for so long. Its emergence has begun to challenge the personal tragedy (individual, medical, deficit) model of disability which informs medical, rehabilitative and broader cultural thinking about disability, wherein disability is individualized and a person's impairment is seen to be either the disability itself[5] or the cause of disability defined as restrictions of activity (Impairment → Disability).[6] The social model is seen by many disabled people to have transformatory potential at the individual as well as the societal level; as Liz Crow (1996: 207) has put it:

> For years now this social model of disability has enabled me to confront, survive and even surmount countless situations of exclusion and discrimination . . . It has enabled a vision of ourselves free from the constraints of disability (oppression) and provided a direction for our commitment to social change. It has played a central role in promoting disabled people's individual self worth, collective identity and political organisation. I don't think it is an exaggeration to say that the social model has saved lives.

It is certainly the case that my own discovery of the social model of disability was liberating at a personal level, and I have a strong sense of the debt that I owe to all of the disabled people who struggled, in their different ways, to bring it into being. The social model is now a touchstone of disability rights politics and Disability Studies in Britain. Mike Oliver's writings have been pioneering: he drew on the UPIAS 'Fundamental Principles' document to formulate the 'social model of disability' (Oliver 1996b). The social model became 'the central concept around which disabled people began to interpret their own experiences and to organise their own political movement' (Oliver 1996c: 26). In the writings of those associated with the disabled people's movement in Britain there is a strong belief that many more social and political gains have been made in recent years by organizations of disabled people informed by the social model perspective than were achieved in previous decades by well-meaning academics and non-disabled people campaigning on behalf of 'the disabled', often through charities or the voluntary sector.

Social barriers

The origins of the social model of disability in the emancipatory struggles of disabled people have been emphasized. This attention to its political origins is very important, not least because it reminds us that ideas do not descend fully formed from the heavens, but are always social products, and because it signals that the social context in which the redefinition of disability occurred played a critical role in shaping the identification of particular social barriers as key. Producing accounts of the history of the British disabled people's movement, and of the role played by particular individuals – for example, Paul Hunt (1966), Vic Finkelstein (1980) and Paul Abberley (1987) – has recently become an important undertaking within Disability Studies (see Shakespeare 1993; Barnes 1996; Campbell and Oliver 1996; Oliver 1996b; 1996c; Campbell 1997). This work indicates that one crucial focus for organizations of disabled people in the 1970s was the poverty commonly experienced by physically impaired people, and the need for decent living standards and employment. The reformulation of disability in the UPIAS 'Fundamental Principles of Disability' document of 1976 was the result of disagreement between it and other disabled people's organizations about political perspectives in relation to employment: 'the struggle to achieve integration into ordinary employment is the most vital part of the struggle to change the organisation of society so that physically impaired people are no longer impoverished through exclusion from full participation' (UPIAS 1976, cited in Oliver 1996b: 25).

> A crucial factor in this coming together, this growing social identification among disabled people, and hence the realisation of a social cause of disability, is that in the last fifty years or so developments in modern technology have made it increasingly possible to employ even the most severely physically impaired people and to integrate us into the mainstream of social and economic activity . . . the alternative to an 'incomes' (or more properly, 'pensions') approach to the particular poverty of disability is to struggle for changes to the organisation of society so that employment and full social participation are made accessible to all people, including those with physical impairments . . . it is necessary to

go forward with the serious struggle for the right to paid, integrated employment and full participation in the mainstream of life.

(UPIAS 1976, cited in Oliver 1996: 23–4)

Given its origins in these crucial economic concerns, it is not surprising that the early formulations concerning the social exclusion of disabled people concentrated on barriers to participation in the labour market. A related issue of great significance was the existence of barriers to independent living following decades of the 'segregation and incarceration' of disabled people in residential institutions and 'special schools'. Self-determination, especially freedom from the control that non-disabled professionals exercised over their lives, was high on the agenda of many disabled activists in the early days of the movement (Campbell and Oliver 1996).

From this initial emphasis on economic concerns and independent living, the social model enabled other socio-structural barriers to come into view and to become foci for political campaigning, often including direct protest action (Barnes 1991; Zarb 1995; Campbell and Oliver 1996; Oliver 1996b). For example: the physical barriers in the built environment and in transport systems which place limits on mobility and access (Zarb 1995; Imrie 1996a; 1996b); the organizational and attitudinal barriers in education which deny equal educational opportunities to disabled children and adults (Barton 1996a; Corbett 1996; Riddell 1996); barriers in the realm of leisure activities (denying access to buildings, or opportunities to participate in cultural events); barriers preventing full participation in civic and political structures and processes (Barnes 1991; Zarb 1995). It became possible to see that people with impairments are socially excluded in every realm of social life, that they are marginalized and denied the basic civil rights that non-disabled people take for granted. Exclusion could also be detected when it presented itself in more subtle, benign or even benevolent forms – in the form of 'help' or assistance: in the health and welfare services, the 'caring professions', the charities, some voluntary organizations, in the behaviour of non-disabled friends, relatives and passers-by (Morris 1991; Swain *et al.* 1993; Thomas 1997; 1998a). These organizations, groups and individuals, although often well-meaning, are almost always guided by the perspective that impairment is a misfortune or a tragedy, that disabled people's problems stem mainly or exclusively from their impairment, that rehabilitation – or restoration to as near as normal functioning as possible – must be the desired goal, and that people with impairment are dependent, limited, objects of pity.

Disabled women constrained by social barriers

This social barriers perspective (Social barriers → Disability), with its foregrounding of socio-structural barriers, can be brought to life by presenting a few extracts from the narratives shared with me by disabled women. The examples used are not isolated – the women's accounts contained many instances of their being constrained by socio-structural barriers. The narratives illustrate that the social model approach represents a very powerful way of making sense of key aspects of many disabled women's life experiences, particularly with respect to education, employment, standards of living, housing and living arrangements, transport and mobility. It should not be forgotten that, for many disabled women and men, the struggle to secure the material means of subsistence, as well as basic civil rights and privileges consonant with living in an advanced industrial society, is uppermost. The political implications are clear: what is required is the removal of social barriers and not the adaptation of individual women to the putatively 'inevitable consequences' of being impaired.

Recounting their personal experiences, Lisa, Denise, Helen and Jane tell us about the social barriers experienced in striving for independent living, self-determination, education and employment, and of the rewards which accrue once (and if) these barriers are overcome. We also get a strong flavour, particularly in Lisa's and Denise's accounts, of the interwoven nature of disability and gender.[7]

Lisa's story is about the disabling nature of the built environment, both houses and workplaces, as well as about prejudicial attitudes among employers. The impact of having an impaired member of the family on household income (giving up paid work, additional costs) is also signalled. Independence is achieved, but not easily.

Lisa, a wheelchair user in her mid-twenties at the time of writing. (Extracts from her letter.)

When I first left the spinal [injury] unit at 19 years of age I had to rely very heavily on my family. At my parents' home there were no facilities for me (bathroom and toilet). So for several months I had a commode and bed baths in my Mum's front room. My Mum gave up work to look after me. It was hard on everyone. A year later I had a shower/toilet room built and the through lounge/dining room was finally blocked off to give me my privacy. I went to college for 2 years which helped me come to terms with my disability. The college I went to as a day student was for people with disabilities. A lot of the other students had more severe disabilities, which made me feel that I was lucky to be able to do as much as I could. When I first started college I needed help to go to the loo. When I left I was fiercely independent. The worst thing about those first few months at home was having to rely on everyone to drive me from A to B. Now seven years down the road, I have my own one bedroom adapted flat, about one and a half miles from my mother's house, handy for dropping off the washing. I work full-time at the [organization of disabled people] . . . and I drive my own hand-controlled car. It's been a struggle to get completely independent but it's worth it, and I wouldn't give it up for anyone. Unless I meet the right partner, but he will have to be pretty special.

Having gone to college, when I left, I was well geared up for work. However finding a job was very difficult, access to the work place was the biggest problem. I remember being asked to go for an interview in an office that was two flights of stairs up and there was no lift. I telephoned to tell them that I used a wheelchair and could not manage any steps. They told me it would not be a problem, as they would arrange for someone to carry me up and down. Were they going to do this twice a day and when I went out for lunch? I think not! They got a nasty letter from me. As getting a job was so difficult I did voluntary work for about a year and through this I got offered a paid job. Unfortunately this lasted only about 6 months as the company went bankrupt. So I went back to voluntary work. Then I got a job selling wheelchairs. Now I've just got a new job for [an organization of disabled people], which has a pretty good salary. It's hard to find work with a decent salary, as a disabled woman you're put at a disadvantage even before the interview. The answer is not to put disabled on the application form, unless you know being disabled is an advantage.

Denise's account testifies to the social barriers faced by disabled people in employment – as manifested in the attitudes and behaviours of non-disabled people in positions of power in the workplace. In her experience as a trade union organizer, disabled women are particularly disadvantaged: sexism interacts with disablism.

Denise, aged 52 at the time of writing. (Extracts from her letters.)

I contracted polio at the age of 2 years old in 1947. It affected my right leg, leaving the leg thin and me with a limp. I also had an operation for a lipoma (a fatty lump) on the lower outside right leg which then left me with an unsightly scar and somewhat mis-shapen leg! Last July I broke my right femur which means I now wear a surgical shoe with caliper and am, hopefully temporarily, on crutches . . .

I worked years ago in a publishing house. When I became an advertisement manager for one of the technical journals I was told that prior to my holding the position, one of the Directors had said when I was suggested for the post, 'But she's got a limp'. It undoubtedly matters in employment. I once overheard a customer, at an exhibition when I changed to another publishing house, say '[The publisher] must be hard up for staff if he has to employ cripples'. Yet the strange thing was, he tried his luck with me one evening when everyone was having drinks at the hotel. I wish I could remember which came first, the spurned approach or the insult. I carry most anger towards that man. I should have hit him! Both times . . .

I work now for [employer] and am also the Convenor for [trade union] Disabled Workers Group. I have found that women are discriminated against doubly when they are disabled. A disabled man gets more help and assistance from management than the women. Equipment, far more flexibility in hours and levels of standards required in their work, are better for men than women. Women who have special needs are largely ignored and refused repeatedly when asking for changes in conditions or new equipment whilst men have higher positions and greater access to better facilities. It appears that when a woman has particular difficulties or has a disability she is seen as creating problems for the employer. When a man has such needs, he is fighting for his career, what guts, what a man! . . .

One member I have assisted has a mobility problem made worse by carrying an enormous weight. Over a period of time management have sent her frequently to the [employer's] own Doctor to see what was causing her problems, instead of accepting the woman HAD problems and trying to assist her with special equipment or a job change. Management have been AWFUL! When we were unable to obtain help from management, we brought PACT in. In an almost tit for tat reaction, they sent her to an arthritic specialist for a report. The specialist wrote back to say that he saw no reason to doubt her statement that she was unable to – for example – file in the lower drawers of a cabinet. The attitude of management has been to almost ostracise her for being bold enough to obtain help from PACT! and have been bordering on obstructive. Another woman employee who suffered from ME needed to have flexible hours. When I consulted with management I was told 'This is not a charity.'

At meetings, most people gripe about the way in which management ignore their problems. I cannot stress enough the almost brutal attitude towards women especially, who are usually at lower grades, by managers. . . . In the seven to eight years I have been Convenor for the Disabled Group, I have never been approached by a disabled man asking for assistance or support. They have been along to the meetings, but all of them were satisfied with their conditions and equipment and attended solely to hear about pensions, the Bill or other such information. The women I have spoken to, experience little or no support and constantly meet with resistance when asking for the same level of support etc.

Helen wrote at length about her life experiences as a partially sighted woman. In the extract below she tells of her school days. Succeeding in education was sometimes an uphill struggle because of the attitudes and behaviours of a few non-disabled individuals.

Helen, aged 59. Helen is partially sighted, as a result of various eye conditions from birth (untreated in the first weeks of life when medical intervention could have helped). In adult life she also developed epilepsy and, later, osteoarthritis. She has had a successful career in teaching (despite numerous barriers along the way).

Most teachers in the [elementary] school were excellent, but one of them was most unsympathetic and rather horrible. She made fun of me because I leant on the desk when I was writing and, to the amusement of a few pupils, threatened to put holly on the desk to stop me. Apart from a few happy months, this woman was my needlework teacher two afternoons a week for four years. My sewing and knitting were horrendous. It did not occur to my teacher that I could not see well enough to do small, even stitches, and that threading a needle was very difficult for me. Instead of helping/encouraging me, she chose to make fun of my pathetic efforts . . .

. . . [At grammar school] most of the staff were very helpful. I owe some of them a great deal. I found it difficult to decipher handwriting of varying size and clarity, especially in French. Several staff were shocked to discover that I could not always read accurately what was on the board, even from the front row . . . In those days few teachers asked children why they had problems with such simple tasks. I don't blame them, they were not trained to teach children with a disability and they had no one to advise them . . .

. . . one insecure young master made life rather difficult for me at times. When he took over my group, he told everyone where to sit, sending tall people to the back. I tried to explain that I needed to sit at the front, but he just would not listen. He told me to keep quiet. He then put some work on the board and told us to get on with it. I put my hand up to tell him that I couldn't read what was on the board, but he told me to put my hand down and get on with my work. When I started to say that I couldn't see, he sent me out of the room, and afterwards gave me detention for arguing . . . [On a later occasion when eye problems had prevented the completion of homework, this master] said that I was a lazy, idle good-for-nothing who had never done a stroke of work since the first year, and that it was common knowledge among the staff that I was always using my eyes as an excuse to get out of work because I was so lazy . . .

The final narrative is Jane's which tells powerfully of the importance of self-determined living and independence. The financial and other barriers to independent living, as well as its rewards, are described.

Jane, aged 49 at the time of interview. Jane has Still's disease, a form of childhood-onset arthritis. She talks here about the years spent in residential care and her struggle to 'get out', to obtain her own accommodation and live independently. A wheelchair user from the age of 17, she now lives in her own home, employs personal assistants who give 24-hour cover, and owns a motor vehicle. (Extract from the interview transcript.)

Jane: . . . then [at age 18] I went to a residential home in —— where I had mixed fortunes, if you like. In the early days, actually, it was a lot better than it was in the latter part, but I spent 24½ years there and the latter part was very unhappy . . . I suppose you can say I went at the right time, if there is such a right time, because the people there were quite intelligent or very intelligent and had lived a, what I call a normal life, you know, some were in the Forces and some had seen the world, and some had been to university and had lived a very wide life and were well educated, so, although some of them were badly disabled, how can I put it, they were, they steered you in the right direction. I think I went at a good time to be moulded because, although I was 18, I was very very green 'cos I'd spent all my life in places where you're told what to do, at boarding schools and hospitals. You have lunch at this hour, you get up at this time, and you go to physio at this time and so on. And I was as green as grass and I suppose they moulded me into quite a tough person, really, as I am. But then, after that, it became International Year of Disabled People. Some had already moved out but it was the start of people moving out into the community or they got married and their partners looked after them and so on, or unfortunately some died through their illnesses and disabilities, and then you got the other end of the spectrum where they were a lot more disabled and either not capable or didn't want to take decisions for themselves about their life and how they wanted to go on, and one thing and another, and so you were rather, I won't say told what to do, but the staff would try and sort of run things, say what you could do and what you couldn't, and unless you were a strong character people seemed quite happy to live by that. I wasn't, and that got worse and worse as more and more badly disabled people came and they didn't really want to be bothered to make decisions and so on. And things got worse and worse and I got more and more unhappy and in those days you were in a very difficult position because you're on benefits and you're not allowed to have savings above a certain amount.

I did try for nine years to get out into a place of my own but the stumbling block every time was that the housing association would only offer you a one-bedroomed place because you're a single person and also there was a huge, huge waiting list, you couldn't guarantee anything. And what they did offer you was so tiny anyway that you couldn't have it. If you have one chance at it you've got to go for, I won't say the biggest and the best, but you've got to really decide what you want and to go for that and not think, well, I'll move into a smaller place and then I'll move into a bigger place later because you might never get the chance . . . I kept getting told we'll not be holding any more, or there's only single things, or you can go on our waiting list, and so on and so on, and everywhere I turned I couldn't get a mortgage because I didn't have enough savings and there wasn't, at the time, any other means really, and so it was very hard. You either sort of rotted away in an unhappy place or you had to have enough money to buy your way out really, that was the basic thing. Anyway, as I say, I tried for nine years, trying everything I knew, everybody I could write to, but without any luck. Anyway, then finally, I don't know whether it was because of my cheek or whether fate took a kindly hand, I used to go to my local football team every Saturday, or every other Saturday, and one of the firms that sponsored them was a financial institution and I just happened to write to them and say 'what could you do for me, if anything, someone who has no savings, has no job and, well, no prospects, no . . . deposit, security?' . . . Anyway, they wrote back. I just thought they'd laugh it out of court, but they didn't. They said, personally, they couldn't help but they were giving a copy of my letter to the —— Building Society, which they must have had dealings with, and that they would get in touch with me, so in due course I got the letter to come and see the manager and explained my position and . . . You see, the thing was, it would have to be the type of mortgage that was, I think they used to call it a retirement mortgage, where they would lend you the money, and just pay on interest only . . . They couldn't help at first, well I'd tried various ones and they couldn't give me more than say 85 per cent or something like that, which wasn't really much good to me 'cos I didn't have enough savings. Anyway, in a way fate took another turn. Through my mother's misfortune – she was an older person and her eyes were going and had various other ailments – she had to move, sell her flat and move into a retirement home so in the selling of her flat she kept enough to pay her expenses in the home and then she gave the three of us in the family a little bit of money. Well, because I'm not allowed to have it handed on a plate, so to speak, she put my share [into this house], she bought my house here along with what I had. I went back to the [building society] and sorted out a mortgage . . . through my mother's misfortune it was my good fortune, but if I hadn't had my mum's money I would still be in the same boat because there's just no way, unless you can work and earn money, you'd not be able to do it, and if you were earning money you wouldn't get benefits anyway so it's a terrible dilemma, you're sort of between a rock and a hard place. But, anyway, now I've sorted it all out about my care. I get help from the government to pay for my own care and I organize it and everything and I've been here six years now and the quality of life and the freedom is just amazing. It's like the other side of the world.

Carol: What are the real differences?

Jane: Well, I think the freedom and choice, and mainly the quality of life, is so much better because you are on a one-to-one. You're not having to share. You're making the decisions. You don't have to be told what time you have to get up, go to bed, or what you're having, or 'sorry, can't come to you it's our coffee break or lunch break', or 'I'm busy now'. You have to wait for the toilet. Now, if you want to go, you go when you say. It's just marvellous to be able to live your own life just as you want, without restrictions.

. . . I did find [it] very hard when I tried [to get my own home] for nine years . . . every time I got a knock back and the door shut again, it was really hard to bring myself to try again and again and again. You think, am I ever going to stop banging my head on the wall? [She mentioned later in the interview that she had contemplated suicide at this time.] But I think when I was at my really most desperate something came about, but as I've said, it's only through mum's misfortune really, and that worries me a lot about people today – there must be many people in my position with no financial backing who are so unhappy but cannot move on, and I really don't know how they would cope with that.

The emergence of critiques of the social model

The broadening of the range of disabling social barriers which can be identified using a social model perspective might appear to have infinite possibilities, but recent debates within the disabled people's movement and Disability Studies indicate that all is not well with the social model. Increasingly, arguments are presented which suggest that the social model – or, more precisely, the analyses advanced in its name – has limits or problems which are either inherent or associated with its partial application.

For some, the social model (or leading social modellists) focuses too heavily, or exclusively, on socio-structural barriers (determining access to life's material necessities) and downplays or ignores the cultural and experiential dimensions of disablism, and this is frequently attributed to the Marxist or materialist perspectives of influential figures such as Mike Oliver, Vic Finkelstein and Colin

Barnes (for example, see critiques by Price 1996; Shildrick and Price 1996; Shakespeare 1997a; Corker 1998a; Corker and French 1999). Another problem which has been identified is that the interests of people who have particular forms of impairment, or pathologized difference, are seen to be ill served or under-represented by the social model because their experiences and needs do not 'fit' the model – for example, people with learning difficulty (Corbett 1996; Warmsley 1997), deafness (Corker 1993; 1998a; Harris 1995) or mental 'illness' (McNamara 1996). A further issue has been the social modellist tendency to ignore or deny the significance of impairment itself, either in disability theory or in terms of its impact on the daily lives of disabled people (Abberley 1987; 1996; 1997; French 1993; Crow 1996; Morris 1996; Hughes and Paterson 1997). Then there are the limits to the social model identified by those who argue that it has worked to marginalize or exclude the experiences of particular groups of disabled people on the basis of gender, sexuality, 'race' or age (or a combination of these). Again, this is usually seen to be either to do with the model's inherent weaknesses or because of its application by men/straight people/white people/young people who tend to construct problems and solutions in their own image: what about disabled women? (see below); disabled gay men, lesbians and bisexuals? (Appleby 1994; Corbett 1994; Shakespeare *et al.* 1996; Shakespeare 1997b); disabled black and minority ethnic people? (Stuart 1993; Begum *et al.* 1994; Priestley 1995; Vernon 1996; 1997); older disabled people or disabled children? (Zarb and Oliver 1992; Kennedy 1996; Morris 1997; Robinson and Stalker 1998).

In resulting debates in Disability Studies and the disabled people's movement there have been calls for the further development, the renewal, the transformation, or even the abandonment, of the social model of disability. Oliver and others have tried to hold the line against some of these criticisms while welcoming others (Oliver 1996b; Finkelstein 1996). At the same time as placing the social model under strain, the debates have also served to greatly enrich Disability Studies, and to make the disabled people's movement more accommodating of 'difference', although many would argue that there is still a long way to go. What is striking, though, is that in the face of another set of critiques of the social model from 'the outside' – for example, by medical sociologists who research disability (Bury 1996a; 1997; Williams 1996a; 1996b; Pinder 1995; 1996; 1997) – there tends to be a closing of ranks in its defence and a careful policing of its boundaries (Barnes and Mercer 1996a; Shakespeare and Watson 1997). This is not surprising given its political history and its significance in the wider disablist social and political environment.

This book has been written with these ongoing debates about the social model of disability, both within Disability Studies and between Disability Studies and medical sociology, in mind. It attempts to engage with and further develop some of the key issues raised in these critiques and debates, and particularly those which relate to, or have a bearing on, matters of gender and the lives of disabled women. I am attempting to contribute to the theorizing of disability as a social phenomenon within Disability Studies, but in a manner which acknowledges the political and conceptual significance of the social model, building on, rather than abandoning, key elements of this model. It would be very easy to forget that the social model of disability has created the space which makes everything else possible. Whatever the weaknesses of the analyses advanced in its name, it *has* 'freed up disabled people's hearts and minds by offering an alternative conceptualisation of the problem. Liberated, the direction of people's personal energies turned outwards to building a force for changing society' (Campbell and Oliver 1996: 20).

The social model of disability should best be thought of as a conceptual point of departure in Disability Studies. It poses rather than answers important theoretical questions about disability: What is the at the root of disabling social barriers? What other social conceptualizations of disability are possible? What are the mechanisms at work in shaping disabled people's experiences? How can the social exclusion of people with impairment be explained? What constitutes impairment? These are large questions, analogous to those seeking explanations for women's oppression, or why black and other minority ethnic groups are discriminated against. Answers will depend on our way of understanding the social world – our theoretical perspective, epistemological framework and ontological starting points (philosophy of what it means 'to be'). As Oliver (1996b: 52) himself reminds us, 'we must not assume that models in general and the social model of disability in particular can do everything; that it can explain disability in totality. It is not a social theory of disability and cannot do the work of social theory'.

Gender

There appears always to have been tension within disabled people's organizations along the gender axis. For example, UPIAS was seen by some disabled women to be problematically masculine in both its organizational nature and its political programme. In the 1970s UPIAS was comprised of men and women who lived in residential institutions, adopted a democratic centralist style of organization, and actively excluded non-disabled and some disabled individuals who did not share its social understanding of disability. Vic Finkelstein, a leading member, argues (in Campbell and Oliver 1996: 67) that its exclusionary and secretive character was a necessity: if the organization opened its doors to everyone then its fragile reformulation of disability in social terms could be destroyed, and the vulnerability of disabled people in institutions meant that they would be open to abuse if they did not keep their critical perspectives under wraps. But, as UPIAS member Maggie Davis put it in an interview in the 1990s:

> From the female perspective I'm sure that there was more than a hint of a hard, not necessarily macho, style in terms of the political and analytical debate; in terms of the dialectic and rigour by which people were expected to defend their positions and stand or fall by them in the process

of self, personal development within the collective ethos. In some senses that has got a very typical masculine political feel to it and I think that it [UPIAS] has to live with that kind of criticism. Later on, when we [the women involved] looked back at the circulars, we saw that fairly clearly. Although we still agreed that it was the right direction that we took.

(Davis, in Campbell and Oliver 1996: 67–8)

From a more critical perspective, the disabled activist Micheline Mason recalls:

At this time [1976–78] there was no organised disability movement in the UK. I believe UPIAS existed, and I was pleased to know that, but having been emotionally and intellectually battered to the floor by one of its leaders, it did not feel it was like anything to which I wanted to belong.

(Mason, in Campbell and Oliver 1996: 52)

Mason's experience parallels a more general 'getting put down by dominating men' experience reported by some women in left-wing political organizations in the late 1960s and 1970s, something which gave an important impetus to the women's liberation movement in those years (Rowbotham 1972; Coote and Campbell 1982). Mason herself was centrally involved in the setting up of a different kind of disabled people's organization at the end of the 1970s, the Liberation Network of Disabled People (LNDP, 1979 to mid-1980s):

LNDP was a woman-led organisation and it embodied female values, although it included men right from the beginning. Through the support groups, and later through the magazine *In from the Cold*, we began to challenge the traditional view of disability as an individual health problem. We challenged the effects of 'internalised oppression', recognised by all marginalised groups as a major 'tool' of the oppressive society; we challenged the conditioned hatred of ourselves and each other as disabled people; we challenged the desire to assimilate; we challenged the denial of 'hidden' disabilities; we challenged the fierce competition between us; we challenged the inability to champion, appreciate and support each other's achievements or thinking (especially when it challenges our own); we challenged the lack of information and understanding about the issues of other oppressed peoples.

(Mason, in Campbell and Oliver 1996: 69)

The importance of 'the personal' is clearly evident in Mason's account of the LNDP, something that the disabled feminist activist and writer, Jenny Morris, has always emphasized. Morris is undoubtedly the most influential writer in Britain on the gendered character of disability and the life experiences of disabled women, and her work is referred to many times in this book. Whilst a staunch supporter of the social model in pursuit of disability rights, Morris has been a critical voice within the disabled people's movement on questions of gender and politics:

Like other political movements, the disability movement in Britain and throughout the world, has tended to be dominated by men both as theoreticians and holders of important organisational posts. Both the movement and the development of a theory of disability have been the poorer for this as there has been an accompanying tendency to avoid confronting the personal experience of disability.

(Morris 1991: 9)

Morris has argued that not only has personal experience been missing from the political agenda of the disabled people's movement, an issue which is explored in some depth in this book, but also that those socio-structural barriers which have been prioritized (such as barriers preventing access to paid work) have tended to be ones of most significance to disabled men (see earlier discussion of this in Deegan and Brooks 1985; Fine and Asch 1988). That is, in addition to the barriers commonly experienced by both disabled men and women, those of particular relevance to many disabled women associated with gendered role responsibilities in the domestic and family domains tend to be ignored:

Disabled women want personal assistance which enables them to look after children, to run a home, to look after parents or others who need help themselves. In contrast, the disabled people's movement has tended to focus on personal assistance which enables paid employment and other activities outside the home.

(Morris 1996: 10)

The concerns of Morris and other disabled women about the invisibility of disabled women's experiences and needs has resulted in the publication in a wide range of scholarly books and papers, as well as autobiographical accounts, poems and narratives, by and about disabled women (Campling 1981; Matthews 1983; Browne *et al.* 1985; Deegan and Brooks 1985; Saxton and Howe 1987; Fine and Asch 1988; Morris 1989; 1991; 1993a; 1995; 1996; Finger 1990; Begum 1992; Driedger and Gray 1992; Mason 1992; Hillyer 1993; Keith 1994; Marris 1996; Wendell 1996; Thomas 1997; 1998a; 1998b; 1999).

As well as being the source of some weighty criticism of the social model of disability and its exponents, this literature tells us something very important: that the experience of disability is always gendered, that disablism is inseparably interwoven with sexism (and racism, and homophobia, and so on). This is not at all to say that disabled women and men have no common ground, no shared experiences of disablism, but that the forms and impacts of disablism are always refracted *in some way* through the prism of gendered locations and gender relations. This is not surprising given that, whether disabled and impaired or not, we all live out lives which are profoundly shaped by the social constructions of gender (which we may, of course, resist and transgress). The gendered nature of disabling experiences was very much confirmed in the letters, self-recorded tapes and interviews transcripts which I gathered for use in this book. Overall, the women's accounts were of lives which were either conventional in terms of gender roles, or were written about and made sense of with reference to the norms of other (non-disabled) women's lives. Many of the women were girlfriends, wives, mothers, grand-mothers and/or informal carers. Some were in happy marriages and non-marital relationships with men, others were in unhappy ones and a few had been divorced. Two talked about the fulfilment they had found in lesbian relationships following years of marriage. Only a few had not experienced sexual or romantic relationships with others. In general, the women who communicated with me were embedded in formal and informal social relationships with individuals and groups which typify 'modern womanhood' at different phases in the life course, and their experience of, and resistance to, disablism cannot be understood independently of the gendered character of their lives – or of the gendered frameworks impacting upon them.

The criticisms made by feminists and other disabled women writers within the disabled people's movement and Disability Studies have certainly not gone unheard, and some male authors have explicitly taken a number of the criticisms on board, often drawing on wider feminist literature in their own writing (see Chapter 4). In fact, the view that disabled women's concerns *continue* to be ignored or downplayed has recently been disputed, for example by Tom Shakespeare (1996b). Shakespeare's own commitment to the import-ance of feminist approaches in Disability Studies suggests that he may well have a point when he says:

> In terms of research and investigation of these issues [gender differences] I would argue that there is a considerable amount of work on disabled women, but hardly any on disabled men (see Campling 1981; Deegan and Brooks 1985; Fine and Asch 1988; Keith 1994; Lonsdale 1990; Morris 1989; Saxton and Howe 1987). Women, working predominantly within feminist contexts have quite rightly explored issues of sexuality, imagery, gender identity and relationships, while men have perhaps con-centrated on issues such as employment, discrimination, housing, income, and other material social issues . . . but generally I think the male domination of traditional disability research has mainly had the effect of leaving gender out of the picture entirely. It seems almost as if disability studies has reproduced the wider split between public and private with which students of gender studies are familiar. The effect of this is that dis-abled men's *experience* is under-represented.
>   (Shakespeare 1996b: 196–7; emphasis added)

I make no apology, however, for adding to the existing literature on dis-abled women's experiences, for reflecting upon debates in Disability Studies in the light of these experiences, and for further examining the implications for disability theory of feminist and other genres of analysis. Many of the issues raised by feminist critics within Disability Studies remain unresolved, reflecting the fact that the development of social theory about disability is still in its infancy.

Shakespeare's observation that Disability Studies has reproduced the split between the public and private is an important one, explored in Chapters 3 and 4. I suggest that this is central to ongoing arguments within the disabled people's movement, and among Disability Studies writers, about the political and theoretical significance of the personal 'experience' of living with disability and impairment, as well as to arguments about the particular forms and mechanisms of oppression which confront disabled people whose social locations differ in connection with their gender, 'race', class, sexuality and age, and according to the nature and social meaning of their impairment(s).

Endings

This chapter has introduced and discussed the social model of disability, highlighting its political rootedness. Disabled women's narratives have been drawn upon to illustrate the importance of social barriers – socio-structural, organizational, environmental and attitudinal – in shaping the lives of disabled people. The gathering criticisms of the social model have also been outlined, as have debates about gender and disability. The scene is now set for the next chapter, which focuses on the contrast between the definition of disability embodied in the social model perspective and that found in the World Health Organization's (WHO) impairment, disability and handicap schema. This, in turn, provides the grounds for a discussion of a disability definitional riddle.

Notes

1 As noted in the Introduction, this book focuses mainly on the British Disability Studies literature. There are, of course, growing Disability Studies literatures (that is, literatures linked with disabled people's organizations) in North America, Australasia and elsewhere. A number of writers have begun to track the distinguishing conceptual and political differences between the British debates and those in other places (see, for example, Barnes 1996; 1997a; Oliver 1996c; Shakespeare 1996a; Gleeson 1997a). For a recent introduction to Disability Studies in the United States, see Davis (1997), which also contains a helpful bibliography.

2 The use of the term 'social construction' can be rather confusing to those familiar with sociological perspectives because what is most commonly meant by social modellists like Oliver is the social creation, or social production, of disability rather than its 'construction' in the discursive, that is, postmodernist or poststructuralist, sense (see Priestley 1998). Social modellists like Oliver mean that disability is socially produced by material social forces and factors, usually referred to as 'social barriers', although ideology is also seen as playing an important role (Oliver 1990; see Chapter 7). As we shall see in later chapters, there is a growing interest in Disability Studies in poststructuralist and postmodernist perspectives.

3 The BCODP was founded in 1981: originally as the British Council of Organisations of Disabled People, now the British Council of Disabled People. It is the national umbrella organization of disabled people in Britain – priding itself on being a democratic, accountable and representative organization. An interesting account of its

formation and development is given in Campbell and Oliver (1996), an overview which openly considers the organization's weaknesses as well as its strengths. Seven national disabled people's organizations (one of which was UPIAS) formed the steering group that constituted the BCODP, but its membership was extended to local organizations in 1982, and to individuals in 1995. For some, the BCODP *is* the disabled people's movement, but for others it is a key part of a wider social movement which includes formal organizations and informal networks such as the disability arts movement. The BCODP represents British disabled people at meetings of the Disabled People's International (DPI).

4 The DPI was formed in 1981. It emerged

> out of the anger of 200 disabled delegates at the two-and-a-half-thousand strong Rehabilitation International (RI) conference in Winnipeg. Disabled delegates were outraged at the decision *not* to ensure disabled people's representation on the IYDP [International Year of Disabled People] organising committee. In protest they walked out, and the now Director of the DPI, Henry Enns, addressed the boycott of disabled people, who came from over thirty counties, saying: 'Do I hear you want to form your own international organisation of disabled people?'
>
> (Campbell and Oliver 1996: 83)

The DPI has held World Congresses in Singapore (1981), the Bahamas (1985), Vancouver (1992), and Sydney (1994). In 1996 I was privileged to be among over 100 disabled women who attended the first *European Conference for Disabled Women* in Munich, on *Self-determined living for women in Europe*, organized by the DPI and Interessenvertretung Selbstbestimmt Leben Deutschland.

5 The equation of impairment and disability is evident in statements like 'her disability is that she is blind'. This conflation is found in Britain in the official documentation associated with the Disability Discrimination Act 1995 where it is stated: 'The Act gives new rights to people who have had a disability which makes it difficult for them to carry out normal day to day activities. The disability could be physical, sensory or mental'.

6 A good example of a contemporary 'medical model' conceptualization of disability is given by Lois Verbrugge (1995: 20):

> Disability refers to the impacts that chronic conditions have on people's ability to act in necessary, typical and personally desired ways in their society. Our attention is on long-term, but not necessarily static, consequences of chronic conditions on physical, mental and social functioning.

Verbrugge's statement is informed by the ICIDH and other definitional schemas (the ICIDH is discussed in Chapter 2). Examples of disability given by Verbrugge (1995: 21) are 'difficulties doing activities of daily life: employment, household management, personal care, hobbies, active recreation, clubs, socializing with friends and kin, childcare, errands, sleep, trips, etc.'. That disability, thus defined, could be caused by social factors and processes that actively exclude people with chronic conditions is simply not considered. The impression given, and the medical research effect, is that the entire focus is on the ways that chronic conditions, or impairments, limit 'people's ability to act' in society. This is not to say that authors like Verbrugge fail to acknowledge that disabled people experience 'social disadvantages' – for example, she notes: 'Not shown . . . is social disadvantage, also known as handicap; it is a genuine experience of persons with disabilities but remains very difficult to measure by objective or even subjective means in surveys'

(Verbrugge 1995: 21). This disadvantage is seen as the effect of disability rather than its cause.

7 See the Introduction for an account of how I came by these disabled women's narratives. It is important to note that in the narratives presented in the book disabled women tended to use the term disability in the lay sense – to mean the impairment itself. In fact, in my press release (discussed in the Introduction), I referred to myself as a woman with 'a disability', but was here using the term 'disability' in its lay sense to signal that I had an impairment. I felt compelled to do this in order to communicate clearly, but I also stated that the research was adopting a 'social model' perspective. Some women used the term 'disability' to mean 'restriction of activity'.

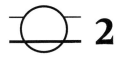 **2**

Defining disability: a definition riddle

Introduction

In contrast to those who adopt a social model definition of disability, some researching in the disability field use a different but authoritative definitional schema: the International Classification of Impairments, Disabilities and Handicaps. This was developed by the epidemiologist, Philip Wood, for the World Health Organization (Wood 1980; see also United Nations 1983).[1]

WHO definitional schema (ICIDH)

Impairment: In the context of health experience, an impairment is any loss or abnormality of psychological, physiological, or anatomical structure or function.

Disability: In the context of health experience, a disability is any restriction or lack (resulting from an impairment) of ability to perform an activity in the manner or within the range considered normal for a human being.

Handicap: In the context of health experience, a handicap is a disadvantage for a given individual, resulting from an impairment or a disability, that limits or prevents the fulfillment of a role that is normal (depending on the age, sex, social and cultural factors) for that individual. (Oliver 1996a: 40–1)

British social modellists reject this schema, arguing that it is a version of the 'medical model' of disability because it sets up a chain of causation wherein impairment causes disability (Impairment → Disability). Handicap is seen to flow, in turn, from disability (Impairment → Disability → Handicap).

This chapter begins with a brief discussion of the ways in which two scholars – one a medical sociologist, Michael Bury, and the other a disabled feminist scholar in Canada, Susan Wendell – use the ICIDH. My purpose is to outline the debates which flow from the clash of definitional approaches, but more particularly to set the scene for discussion of a definitional riddle about disability which I struggled with for some time, and hope to have resolved. The resolution assists in two ways: first, in breaking through one of the stalemates in contemporary debates about the meaning and causes of disability, especially debates between social modellists and medical sociologists; and second, because it allows me to argue for a more clearly expressed *social relational* definition of disability. This, in turn, facilitates the uncovering of what I will call *impairment effects*, without resurrecting the idea that 'impairment causes disability'. This lays the foundations for the analyses in subsequent chapters.

A medical sociologist on disability

Michael Bury, who has defended the use of the ICIDH schema in his research on chronic illness and disability, has recently described the British medical and social policy context in which it emerged (Bury 1996a; 1996b; 1997). His account testifies to the real consequences of definitions in terms of the way they come to inform state legislation and the pattern of welfare provision. He noted that the ICIDH definitions were an attempt to clarify the rather confusing terminology which had been used in the first piece of government-sponsored national research on 'impairment and handicap'. This was the British Office of Population Censuses and Surveys (OPCS) study by Amelia Harris *et al.* (1971a; 1971b):

> This showed, for the first time, the extent of impairment in Britain, and suggested that just under 4% of the population aged 16–64 and just under 28% of the population over the age of 65 suffered from some form of impairment [Harris *et al.* 1971a]. Interestingly, gender differences were noted, with twice the level of impairment in women compared with men . . .
>
> (Bury 1996a: 19)

Bury noted that Harris *et al.*'s research was associated with the passing of the 1970 Chronically Sick and Disabled Persons Act in Britain, which obliged local authorities to estimate and 'meet the needs' of disabled people. The ICIDH schema, with its definition of disability as restriction of activity caused by impairment, was subsequently used in Jean Martin's OPCS disability study commissioned in 1984 (Martin *et al.* 1988; Bruce *et al.* 1991).[2] This study involved several surveys carried out between 1985 and 1988. Bury (1996a: 119) notes that the study was designed 'to inform a review of social security in the disability field and pave the way for such benefits to be based less on medical assessment'; the policy consequences were the advent of the Disability

Living Allowance (DLA) and the Disability Working Allowance (DWA) (Bury 1997: 29). In terms of the prevalence and age distribution of disability (as defined by the ICIDH):

> The survey showed that of six million people living in Great Britain with at least one form of disability, based on the relatively low threshold used in the survey, almost 70 per cent of disabled adults were aged 60 and over, and nearly half were aged 70 and over (Martin *et al.* 1988: 27). The very old emerge as those most likely to be affected, with 63 per cent of women and 53 per cent of men over the age of 75 being disabled. When severity is taken into account, the very old predominate, with 64 per cent of adults in the two highest categories aged 70 or over and 41 per cent aged 80 or over (ibid). Given that women significantly outnumber men at this age, the gender imbalance in chronic illness is clearly of note.
>
> (Bury 1997: 120)

Bury acknowledged that the ICIDH schema is not without its problems, including the following:

> At the research level, it had long been recognised that the definition of disability, unlike disease, was less categorical and more 'relational' in character. It was pointed out that the term disability was conceptually 'slippery' and difficult to pin down (Topliss 1979), and involved complex interactions between the individual and the social environment. Moreover, the boundaries between impairment, disability and handicap were recognised as less than clear cut in everyday settings, and difficult to operationalise in research, even though the distinctions remained important in directing attention to different planes of experience.
>
> (Bury 1996a: 20)

Nevertheless, Bury saw merit in the schema and what he has called a 'socio-medical model of disabling illness'. In particular, the schema assists in 'focusing on important aspects of experience' (Bury 1997: 138) and, importantly for him, highlights a causal link between chronic illness and what he understands disability to mean: 'restriction or lack of ability to perform activities'.

> The predominance of chronic illness as a cause of disability is also noted in the OPCS study. Many of the disorders associated with later life, especially arthritis and hearing loss (the former helping to explain much of the gender difference in disability rates) were the most frequent causes of disability. This underlined the long-term trend . . . away from disabilities caused by trauma and medical conditions in early life towards those associated with illness in later life. Though not all forms of disability are caused by chronic illness, most are.
>
> (Bury 1997: 120)

With critiques by social modellists in mind, Bury has argued that sociological research which built on work within the socio-medical tradition *has*, among other things, recognized and explored handicap – the disadvantaging social and material consequences of disability. He has recently acknowledged that, 'as has been argued, some aspects of disability are clearly a function of social expectations and the impact of social structure' (Bury 1997: 137), but goes on to say that Oliver's social model formulation presents an 'over-socialised', 'reductionist' and 'unidimensional' picture of the processes involved:

> Such an approach [Oliver's] can easily gloss over social realities and reduce complexities of individual and social responses to a unidimensional view of disability. In particular it can systematically miss the point . . . that the vast majority of disabled people suffer from chronic illness.
>
> (Bury 1997: 138)

Bury also sees dangers in the 'political correctness' demanded of academics by some in the disabled people's movement, particularly in connection with disability research, because in his view this has the effect of proscribing certain types of disability research, thus limiting academic freedom (Bury 1996a; 1996b). I will return to Bury's definitional stance later in this chapter (for further discussion of the differences in perspective between medical sociologists and those in Disability Studies, see Chapter 8).

Susan Wendell's definitional approach

In an interesting discussion of the ICIDH schema the Canadian-based feminist scholar, Susan Wendell (1996), who identifies herself as disabled, also considers the problem of the 'relative' nature of its definition of disability, and she too notes the connection between definitions of disability, social policy and everyday meanings: 'Definitions of disability officially accepted by government bureaucracies and social service agencies determine people's legal and practical entitlement to many forms of assistance, where assistance is available' (Wendell 1996: 11–12). Thus, along with medical diagnoses of illness and impairment, official definitions of disability 'legitimate' particular social meanings, statutes and roles, and these have profound consequences for people who do or do not fit the 'disabled person' criteria.

On the relativity problem with the ICIDH definition of disability, Wendell observes that the schema includes statements which make universalist claims like 'in the manner or within the range considered normal for a human being'. Wendell points out that there are no such universal norms of human structure, function or physical ability in the sense that activities which are 'the norm' in one society may not be in another; both are socially relative:

> Good definitions of impairment and disability should recognize that normal (i.e., unimpaired) physical structure and function, as well as normal (i.e., non-disabled) ability to perform activities, depend to some extent on the physical, social, and cultural environment in which a person is living, and are influenced by such factors as what activities are

necessary to survival in an environment and what abilities a culture considers most essential to a participant.

(Wendell 1996: 22)

In Wendell's view, this difficulty also extends to the ICIDH definition of handicap:

> Because that definition refers to 'a role that is normal, depending on age, sex, social and cultural factors, for that individual', the definitions imply that women can be disabled, but not handicapped, by being unable to do things which are not part of the 'normal' roles of women in their societies. Thus, for example, if it is not considered essential to a woman's role in a given society that she be able to read, then a blind woman who is not provided with education in Braille or good alternatives to printed material is not handicapped by that lack of assistance, according to these definitions. In general, where the expectations for women's participation in social and cultural life are considerably lower than they are for men, disabled women's opportunities will be severely constrained . . .

(Wendell 1996: 17)

In the light of these problems, Wendell decided to adapt the ICIDH schema for her own purposes rather than reject it wholesale, using the term 'disability' to refer to 'any lack of ability to perform activities to an extent or in a way that is either necessary for survival in an environment or necessary to participate in some major aspect of life in a given society' (Wendell 1996: 23). Importantly for my argument below, she retains the ICIDH idea that disability is about restriction of activity. She refers to her analysis of disability as 'social constructionist', but goes on to say that disability has biological, social and experiential components: 'I call the interaction of the biological and the social to create (or prevent) disability "the social construction of disability"' (Wendell 1996: 35). Thus, restrictions of activity are seen as caused by the interaction of social, biological and other factors. Within this framework, she asserts that the social causes of disability play the key role, and that disabled people are socially oppressed.

Wendell outlines a range of ways in which social factors, cultural processes *and* impairment cause disability. The social and cultural processes include the following:

> disability is socially constructed by such factors as social conditions that cause or fail to prevent damage to people's bodies; expectations of performance; the physical and social organization of societies on the basis of a young, non-disabled, 'ideally shaped', healthy adult male paradigm of citizens; the failure or unwillingness to create ability among citizens who do not fit the paradigm; and cultural representations, failures of representation, and expectations.

(Wendell 1996: 45)

This demonstrates that Wendell's ICIDH-type definition of disability allows her to take account of the 'causative' role played by a wide range of social factors which most British social modellists would ignore because they would be seen to be causes of impairment rather than disability (Social factors → Impairment → Disability). Examples are: environments and hostile acts between people that damage people's bodies (most obviously, wars, violent crimes, physical and sexual abuse, rape); patterns of distribution of basic resources (water, food, shelter) which may damage the health of some within the society; hazardous working conditions; and medical care, treatments and practices – among them technologies for keeping sick or impaired bodies alive when they would not previously have survived, and medical practices that harm – see also Abberley's (1987; 1996; 1997) work on the social creation of impairment, discussed in Chapter 7.

The challenge

In their different ways, Bury and Wendell pose a challenge to the social model of disability concerning the relationship between impairment and disability: how can social modellists really deny that 'restrictions of activity' – disability – are, in part, *caused by* illness and impairment? Surely it is obvious that *some* restrictions of activity are caused by limited physical, sensory or intellectual functioning? How can Oliver (1996a) say that disability is wholly and exclusively caused by social barriers? In Britain, debate between medical sociologists and Disability Studies theorists on this question seems to have reached something of a stalemate, with on the one side medical sociologists like Bury arguing that disability is caused, in large measure, by illness and impairment, and on the other side social modellists like Oliver strongly defending the social model by both reiterating the UPIAS definition of disability (given in Chapter 1) and asserting that disability – the restrictions of activity experienced by people with impairment – is wholly and exclusively socially caused (Barnes and Mercer 1996a).

This debate became more complicated when critical voices began to emerge *within* the British disabled people's movement and Disability Studies arguing that the social model did not allow room for the acknowledgement of the role played by impairment and illness in restricting activity and in determining the life experiences of disabled people (Abberley 1987; 1997; Morris 1991; 1996; French 1993; Crow 1996; Hughes and Paterson 1997). For example, Jenny Morris (1991: 10) has said:

> there is a tendency within the social model of disability to deny the experience of our own bodies, insisting that our physical differences and restrictions are entirely socially created. While environmental barriers and social attitudes are a crucial part of our experience of disability – and do indeed disable us – to suggest that this is all there is to it is to deny the personal experience of physical and intellectual restrictions, of illness, of the fear of dying.

Similarly, Sally French, a disabled activist and scholar, has drawn on her own experiences as a visually impaired person to note that some restrictions on her activity *are* 'caused by' her impairment, cannot be wholly explained by the presence of disabling social barriers, and would remain whatever social arrangements might pertain:

> While I agree with the basic tenets of [the social] model and consider it to be the most important way forward for disabled people, I believe that some of the most profound problems experienced by people with certain impairments are difficult, if not impossible, to solve by social manipulation.
>
> (French 1993: 17)

In subsequent work, French (1994) has argued that four factors play a key role in shaping a person's experience of impairment: the point in life at which the impairment is acquired; the relative visibility of an impairment; the comprehensibility of the impairment to others; and the presence or absence of illness (cited in Priestley 1998: 84).

The definitional riddle

For some time I was puzzled by these debates, and was aware that something was eluding me. I was strongly drawn to the UPIAS definition of disability (repeated below), and agreed with the recasting of disability in social terms, but this apparently meant that I had to adopt a position that restrictions of activity are exclusively caused by social factors, and that illness and impairment are not disabling. On the other hand, I could also see that there was much in the arguments advanced by Bury and Wendell, as well as by Morris, French, and Crow among others, that made sense – I could think of plenty of instances where physical, sensory and intellectual states (impairment, illness) could directly cause restrictions of activity irrespective of social arrangements and so be 'disabling'. I was stuck in a riddle. *Disability is about restrictions of activity which are socially caused. That is, disability is entirely socially caused. But some restrictions of activity are caused by illness and impairment. Thus some aspects of illness and impairment are disabling. But disability has nothing to do with impairment.* Eventually I solved the puzzle: the problem is rooted in the residual equation of 'disability' with 'restrictions of activity' in some social modellist writings. This requires more detailed explanation which I shall now attempt to set out.

The social relational and the property definitions of disability

In discussions about the social model of disability there is an assumption made by its advocates, defenders and critics (whether from outside or within Disability Studies) that everyone is interpreting the new social model definition of disability to mean the same thing. In fact, it is actually interpreted in one of two quite different ways: two social definitions of disability are operationalized and frequently conflated. There is a common slippage from one to the other, sometimes even within a single paper. This realization meant that when reading the work of those debating definitions, I began to distinguish carefully which of the two social definitions was being operationalized and/or attributed to others at any one time.[3]

The social relational approach

The first variant is what I will call a *social relational* definition of disability, most clearly expressed in the UPIAS position: disability is 'the disadvantage or restriction of activity caused by a contemporary social organisation which takes no or little account of people who have . . . impairments and thus excludes them from the mainstream of social activities' (UPIAS 1976, cited in Oliver 1996b: 22). Here, disability is *a social relationship between people* (Disability = the social imposition of restrictions of activity on impaired people). In the UPIAS formulation, disability expresses an unequal social relationship between those who are impaired and those who are non-impaired, or 'normal', in society. Thus, in the same way that the concept of patriarchy refers to the relationship of male ascendancy over women, so the concept of disability refers to the relationship of ascendancy of the non-impaired over the impaired. Disability, like patriarchy, is a form of social oppression.[4]

The concept of disability is unhinged from the abstract formulation, 'restrictions of activity', and given an altogether different and more weighty meaning, a meaning which also suggests that disability has historical and spatial specificity. Disability becomes a particular form of unequal social relationship which manifests itself through exclusionary and oppressive practices – *disablism* – at the interpersonal, organizational, cultural and socio-structural levels in particular societal contexts. The challenge is to understand why and how disability takes particular forms in particular contexts. Like sexism or racism, disablism can operate consciously or unconsciously, directly or indirectly, and may be acted out in social interactions between individuals or may be institutionalized and embedded in organizational structures and statutes. Many 'restrictions of activity' result.

This social relational reframing of disability is the one that I favour and develop in this book; it is this definitional approach which needs to be utilized more consistently as the starting point in theoretical work on disability.

The property approach

The second definition of disability in circulation among social modellists is actually a variant of the ICIDH definition, but without the parenthetical reference to 'resulting from impairment'. Here, disability is *a property of the person with impairment*: 'a disability is any restriction or lack . . . of ability to perform an activity' (Disability = restrictions of activity experienced by people with impairment). Disability is then causally attributed to social factors. A two-stage proposition is involved: disability is restricted activity of the person (not being able to do things); and it is caused by social barriers. This *property* version of the definition of disability is widely used, or fallen back upon, within the disabled people's movement, but it represents an incomplete break with the ICIDH schema – it hangs on to the notion that disability consists of individuals' 'restrictions of activity', then simply reverses the direction of causality so that social . factors are seen as 'causing' these, instead of impairment or chronic illness. If disability is understood in this property sense then, by implication, disability is in existence wherever impaired people experience restricted activity – it is then a question of looking for the social barriers. As a consequence, disability becomes a ubiquitous, transhistorical phenomenon, likely to be found in all times and places.

Conflation

This disentangling of these two social model conceptualizations of disability may at first sight seem to be an exercise in hair-splitting, but they do invest the concept 'disability' with very different meanings. A lack of clarity about these matters has served to set up false antitheses in debates within Disability Studies, and between Disability Studies and medical sociology. A key problem is that in many discussions and disagreements about definitions in Britain, the two quite different ways of conceptualizing disability in the name of the social model – first, as an unequal social relationship between impaired and non-impaired people; and second, as a property of the person with impairment (restricted activity) which is then attributed to social factors – tend either to be used as if they were interchangeable or to be conflated. This is at the root of the riddle.

For example, in his rejection of the social model of disability, Bury (1996a; 1997) interprets it in the second, property, sense – not least because he uses the ICIDH schema in his own research. He believes social modellists to be saying that *all* restrictions of activity experienced by people with impairment are socially caused. He can therefore quite easily dismiss the social model by asserting that illness and impairment *obviously* cause some (in his view, most) restrictions of activity, and that the social model is therefore 'oversocialised', 'reductionist' and 'unidimensional' in character. In doing this, Bury is not required to engage with a social relational definition of disability – one which, in my opinion, sociologists would have more difficulty in rejecting. In reply to Bury, Oliver (1996a) invokes the UPIAS (and DPI) social relational definition of disability *and* gives credence to the property definition of disability by asserting that disability resides in restrictions of activity experienced by people with impairments, and that these are entirely caused by social barriers – so that 'disablement is nothing to do with the body' (Oliver 1996a: 42). To add to the confusion, Oliver (1996a: 42) also notes that 'some illnesses may have disabling consequences' (how can illness not be a cause of 'disability' and yet be 'disabling'?).

The effect of the conflation is that the UPIAS definition of disability has come to be extended to mean that *all* disadvantages and restrictions of activity experienced by people with impairment are caused by social factors – an unhelpful universalistic interpretation of the UPIAS stance. This extended, or hybridized, interpretation of the UPIAS definition is now in common usage. That is, the social relational proposition that disability is the social imposition of restrictions of activity on impaired people has become the proposition that *all restrictions of activity experienced by people with impairment are caused by social barriers.*

Easy target

Once the social relational UPIAS definition comes to have an extended, universalistic, interpretation, and impairment is said to have nothing to do with causing 'disability' because it has nothing to do with causing 'restrictions of activity', it is fairly easy to reject to the resulting 'social model', as Bury does, by looking for examples which show that *some* restrictions of activity *are* directly caused by impairment (trauma, illness). 'Debate' then becomes a game of spotting instances where one can identify the cause of a restriction of activity as being either impairment-based or socially caused. The flip side is that an analysis like Susan Wendell's is rejected by social modellists because disability is not seen as entirely socially caused.

To return to the points made by Jenny Morris, Sally French and others within Disability Studies, it now becomes evident that their objection is actually to this universalistic version of the UPIAS definition of disability. Their problem with the social modellist denial of a role for impairment in causing restrictions of activity (and other effects) would not have arisen if disability were understood in a social relational sense, because it would then be entirely permissible to acknowledge that there are also impairment effects that restrict activity and impact in important ways upon the lives of impaired people. It is to impairment effects that I now turn.

Impairment effects

It is important to understand that the UPIAS social relational approach, that disability is the social imposition of restrictions of activity on impaired people, does *not* assert that *all* disadvantages or restrictions of activity experienced by people with impairment constitute 'disability'. That some restrictions of activity may be directly associated with, or 'caused by', having a physical, sensory or intellectual impairment (not being able to do certain things because of the absence of a limb or the presence of chronic pain or fatigue, for example) is not ruled out – it is just that these are not 'disabilities'. Thus, the fact that I cannot hold a spoon or a saucepan in my left hand is an effect of my impairment and does not constitute disability in the social relational sense. However, this restriction of activity may become the marker for *other* restrictions of activity which do constitute disability if, for example, people in positions of power decide that because I cannot perform such actions then I am unfit to be a paid care worker, or a parent, and should therefore be denied employment, or the privilege of becoming a mother. In this case, the disability resides in the denial of rights, or the refusal to assist me in overcoming functional limitations, for example, by allowing me to do things in an unconventional way, or by helping me to access instruments and technologies which would compensate for not being able to hold things 'normally'. Forthwith, I will use the term *impairment effects* when referring to the restrictions of activity which are associated with being impaired but which are not disabilities in the social relational sense. Impairment effects *may* become the medium of disability in particular social relational contexts. Care must always be taken, of course, not to mistake impairment effects for what are, in fact, disabilities.

The distinction being made between disability and impairment effects cannot be mapped on to the familiar social/biological or cultural/natural dualisms – with disability being about the *social* or cultural and impairment effects being about the effects of the *biological* or the *natural*. As stated in the Introduction, and discussed in some detail in Chapters 6 and 7, impairment and impairment effects should not be naturalized, or dealt with as pre-social 'biological' phenomena. They are profoundly bio-social, that is, shaped by the interaction of biological and social factors, and are bound up with processes of socio-cultural naming. Finally, from the point of view of disabled individuals, 'lived experience' is such that disability and impairment effects interact, and meld together in a holistic fashion. This means that, in a society in which the dominant discourses attribute all restrictions of activity to the 'tragedy' of impairment, it is of great political significance to conceptually separate out disability from impairment effects. In my view, this is the achievement of the social relational conceptualization of disability pioneered by those who formulated the UPIAS definitional approach.

Of course, Oliver and others might argue that the concept of impairment effects lets the medical model in by the back door by conceding too much to the view that impairment itself does play some role in restricting the activity of people with impairment. I would argue that the greater danger lies in allowing the confusion over social definitions of disability to persist such that, on the one hand, medical sociologists and others can continue to ignore the challenge posed by a social relational reframing of the concept of disability, whilst, on the other hand, Disability Studies writers and activists get sidetracked into having to argue for an acknowledgement of the existence and significance of impairment effects. Further, I would suggest that whilst the priority within Disability Studies is to undertake theoretical work and empirical research on disability, defined in the social relational sense, there is also a need to develop a theoretical understanding of impairment and impairment effects *per se*, and to explore the interaction between disability and impairment effects in people's lives.

Endings: back to a social relational definition of disability

The tendency to conflate the social relational and the property definitional approaches in the name of the social model of disability is unfortunate because it blocks both the development of a fuller understanding of the social relational character of disability in the UPIAS sense, and the gaining of a clearer understanding of the nature and limits of impairment effects. Indeed, the conflation tends to short-circuit the opportunity to understand many disabled people's lives as shaped in fundamental ways by the *interaction* of disability and impairment effects – especially the lives of those whose impairments carry the medical diagnostic labels signifying chronic illnesses and/or degenerative conditions.

The social relational conceptualization of disability changes the meaning of disability itself rather than simply switching attention to the social as opposed to biological causes of restrictions of activity. I have argued that it only confuses matters to assert, as some social modellists do, that the UPIAS definition means that '*all* restrictions of activity are socially caused'. Any attempt to eclipse impairment effects by arguing that all restrictions of activity experienced by impaired people have 'nothing to do with the body' seems to me to be a hopeless quest, and it only wastes time to get embroiled in debates about whether or not impairment causes restrictions of activity, or whether or not the social model denies a role for impairment effects in disabled people's lives.

In my view, the strength of the UPIAS definition of disability is precisely its reformation of the concept of disability as a social relational category, and it is this which holds out the best hope for the development of a social theory, or a sociology, of disability. The challenge becomes one of understanding and explaining the particular form of oppressive social relationship between those who are designated 'impaired' and those designated 'non-impaired' (or 'normal'), that is, the relationship which constitutes disability. It means that the key theoretical questions flagged up in Chapter 1 can be further refined: How is the social relationship which constitutes disability generated and sustained within social systems and cultural formations, and why does it exist? How does this social relationship operate and manifest itself?[5] From my materialist feminist theoretical perspective, disability – like other forms of oppression associated with gender, 'race' and so on – is bound up with the level of development of the productive forces, the social relations of production and reproduction, and the socio-cultural and ideological formations which are found in particular societies. This perspective is explored in subsequent chapters. Important descriptive and explanatory work has already been done within Disability Studies on features of disablism, but I would suggest that a definitive and explicit break with the property and hybridized versions of the social model definition of disability would assist greatly.

Arguing for a consistent usage of a social relational definition of disability is only the beginning. In the next chapter I want to consider dimensions of disability, of disablism, which tend to be obscured in the work of many social modellists because the emphasis has been on restrictions *of activity* and material disadvantage: on socially imposed barriers and limits to *what we can do*. What has been obscured are the social barriers and limits to our psycho-emotional well-being, and to our sense of *who we are* or *who we can be*.

Notes

1 It is important to note that the ICIDH, and its usage in government-sponsored disability research, marks a break with the 'Impairment = Disability' equation, or with the 'disability as loss of faculty' perspective which had underpinned the war pensions and industrial injuries schemes in twentieth-century Britain. With the ICIDH, disability becomes the *impact* of impairment on activities which are considered 'usual' in social functioning. In Wood's schema, the meaning of disability is reformulated, or clarified, so that attention could be given to what he saw as the everyday social consequences of impairment for the person. Pre-existing ideas about disability were thus challenged. The ICIDH (or variants of it) is now widely used in medical, rehabilitative, health services, and related research (although the 'Disability = Impairment' idea is still to be found). In occupational therapy and physiotherapy, in particular, the emphasis is now on 'activities of daily living', with the development of measures to assess this – for example, the widely used Barthel Index.

2 For a critique of this OPCS study from a social modellist perspective, see Oliver (1990); Abberley (1992); for Bury's response see Bury (1996a; 1996b).

3 Actually, matters are further muddled by the fact that it is not uncommon in the British Disability Studies literature to find replications of the lay usage of the term 'disability'. That is, authors sometimes slip back into speaking of 'the disability' when they actually mean the impairment itself. Old habits die hard. In the North American Disability Studies literature, on the other hand, the redefinition of the term 'disability' has not occurred in the same way as in Britain, and it is commonplace to see the term being used as a substitute for the 'impairment' (on the debate about terminology in the USA, see Zola 1993).

4 This is, of course, to state the case very bluntly, and there are many refinements which need to be made in following this line of analysis, for at least three reasons. First, there is no fixed boundary between being non-impaired and impaired since this is bound up with socio-cultural meanings and does not rest on supposed biological givens, that is, 'normalities' and 'abnormalities'. Second, one's inclusion among 'the impaired' is a matter of degree and/or may be contingent. Third, there is no fixed boundary between the non-impaired and the impaired in another sense – individuals move from the former into the latter category if they acquire what are socio-culturally identified as impairments during their lifetime (which is, of course, common with advancing age); oppressors thus become the oppressed.

5 This is something I have tried to do, in a small way, in my research on disabled mothers (Thomas 1997; 1998a; Thomas and Curtis 1997).

3

Disability and the social self

Introduction

In the previous chapter I argued that a social relational definition of disability should be the starting point for the development of a social theory (or theories) of disability. This chapter suggests that it is also necessary to broaden the social relational focus from the current one on the social imposition of restrictions of activity on impaired people. By this I mean that other dimensions of socially imposed restrictions should move more centre-stage within Disability Studies, those which operate to shape personal identity, subjectivity or the landscapes of our interior worlds – and work along psychological and emotional pathways. Hereafter, these will be referred to in shorthand as the *psycho-emotional dimensions of disablism*.[1] To put it another way, the focus should include not only a concern for what 'we *do*' and 'how we *act*' (are prevented from doing and acting) as disabled people, but also a concern for 'who we *are*' (are prevented from being), and how we feel and think about ourselves. In everyday life, the impact of disablism along these two dimensions – shaping how we act and who we are – is interactive and compounding.

There is, of course, a huge literature in social psychology and psychiatry on the 'psychological problems' faced by disabled people. It is not my intention to review this literature here, not least because it has been well critiqued by others in Disability Studies (see, for example, Asch and Fine 1988; Finkelstein and French 1993; Shakespeare and Watson 1997). In brief, this literature is characterized by a medically informed 'personal tragedy' perspective on disability, and is noted for its naturalizing of impairment and disability. It is preoccupied with issues of individual adjustment to, coping with and making the best of, the misfortune of 'being disabled'. Personality factors are seen as crucial to a successful or unsuccessful adjustment at the level of the individual. In contrast, I am highlighting the psycho-emotional as a dimension of disablism – arising out of oppressive social relationships – which require for their resolution not 'adaption' of individual people with impairment to their 'misfortune', but changes in the socio-cultural fabric.[2]

Broadening the social relational definition of disability: beyond 'doing'

It is important to stress that I am not referring here to psycho-emotional · effects which are the immediate consequences of impairment, for example, being in pain or experiencing fatigue, physical discomfort, somatically engendered anxiety or disorientation. These psycho-emotional impairment effects are significant, however, since they play a part in many disabled people's lives, and have to be understood in social and not just biological terms.[3] Thus, in the same way that disability both restricts activity and has psycho-emotional dimensions, so too do impairment effects. This chapter is concerned with the psycho-emotional dimensions *of disability*. I am suggesting that as well as the social barriers which are experienced as externally imposed 'restrictions of activity' as currently recognized by social modellists – for example, not being able to obtain employment, appropriate housing, the resources for independent living, and so on – there are also social barriers which erect 'restrictions' within ourselves, and thus place limits on our psycho-emotional well-being: for example, feeling 'hurt' by the reactions and behaviours of those around us, being made to feel worthless, of lesser value, unattractive, hopeless, stressed or insecure.

I am not suggesting, however, that disabled people are simply passive recipients or 'victims' of this disablism. On the contrary, they exercise agency and resist. In some cases simply staying alive and not surrendering to thoughts of suicide is an expression of resistance, in other cases resistance is fuelled by a belief in the value of the self and the refusal to think of one's life as a 'tragedy'.[4] Some find the strength to resist through a religious faith, others by meeting with people in similar circumstances, or in the collective political struggles of disabled people for civil rights. Yet others find it in the empowerment they experience when involving themselves in disability arts. The point is that there is always a need to resist – an ever present requirement to reforge resistance strategies. For most disabled people, though, there are times in their lives when disablism succeeds in severely undermining their psycho-emotional well-being.

Barriers on the outside, inside

This 'inner world' dimension of disablism is closely bound up with socio-cultural processes which generate negative attitudes about impairment and disability, and sustain prejudicial meanings, ideas, discourses, images and stereotypes. These impact upon disabled people in diverse ways and can lodge themselves in their subjectivities, sometimes with profoundly exclusionary consequences by working on their sense of personhood and self-esteem. The agents, or 'carriers', of this disablism may be people 'close' to us: husbands, wives, partners, parents, other family members; or they may be individuals with whom we have direct contact, such as health and social care professionals and workers. They also include unknown individuals and disembodied others in the media and wider culture. Disabled people may have been (and perhaps continue to be) agents of this disablism themselves – promulgating negative attitudes about people with impairments before acquiring their own impairments and disabilities.

This disablism can indirectly act to 'restrict activity': 'I won't apply for this job because, whilst I know I'm capable of doing it, I just don't have the confidence to face people's negative reactions to me and my body'. My argument is that such 'personal' consequences of living in a disabling society should not be thought of as either the 'natural' consequence of 'being impaired' (as in the medical model of disability), or as the 'private troubles' of living with disability which are not really of intellectual or political concern to the disability movement (as in versions of the social model which ignore 'the personal', discussed in Chapter 4). Rather, they should be thought of as part and parcel of disability itself, and an important dimension of disablism in society which needs to be challenged.

This is not at all to deny the importance of restrictions on one's ability to *do* things, to act in the social world. Such restrictions are central to many disabled people's material conditions of life. However, it is to assert that this is not all there is to disablism; there are additional, often intangible, dimensions to the social exclusion of people with impairments, which may in turn have behavioural and other practical consequences. These psycho-emotional dimensions of disability are just as 'social' in origin as are the 'restrictions of activity' experienced in the labour market, in transportation, in education, in housing, in leisure pursuits, or wherever. Thus, spending most of one's time at home because one feels ashamed of a facial disfigurement, or not telling a boyfriend or girlfriend about one's epilepsy for fear of a hostile reaction, are also manifestations of disablism alongside its more familiar consequences: not being short-listed for a job, or not being able to get one's wheelchair into a shop.

Experiencing the psycho-emotional dimensions of disablism

In the daily lives of disabled people, the accumulated consequences of numerous encounters with disablism mean that it is difficult, sometimes impossible, to prize apart the impact and effects of this or that dimension, or feature, of disability. In addition, the experience of disability is mixed in with the experience of living with impairment effects (which also restrict activity and have psycho-emotional aspects), together with the consequences of living out lives which are simultaneously gendered, 'raced', sexed, aged and so forth. 'Lived experience' is thus rich and multi-dimensional, where already complex features of impairment effects and disability meld together with other facets of our social identities. Nevertheless, in the accounts of their lives shared with me by disabled women, it is possible to identify narratives which are illustrative of the psycho-emotional dimensions of disablism (see also, Thomas 1997; 1998b; 1999). These first-person accounts illustrate what I mean by the psycho-emotional dimensions of disability much more powerfully than can a relatively abstract academic discussion, and, once again, they underline the gendered nature of disability. I include just a few examples here.

Dorothy's narrative tells of the painful feelings of rejection which can accompany a sudden relocation in the world of the impaired. Non-disabled people with whom one was once close frequently melt away, leaving self-doubt and sadness.

Dorothy, in her late fifties or early sixties (age not given). Dorothy had a very serious shoulder, neck and spine injury whilst working as a nurse some years previously, and is now a wheelchair user. Her life has changed very dramatically, as have her feelings about herself. (Extract from her letter.)

I am married, and have [adult] sons . . . Only one sister [of many siblings] came to help and she lasted 3 days! She was unable to accept me and she still, after [all this time], will not accept my wheelchair. The rest of my [siblings] do not get in touch, not even a card at Christmas, at first I did not accept this as we had been a so-called 'close knit' family.

My husband works abroad and was on leave when my second operation was due. I had seen the surgeon, and been told to go home and discuss with my family whether to have the operation or not, because the 'odds' against a successful operation were very high. I was told that I could be paralysed from the neck down, or even lose my life. They did not hold out a great deal of hope for me being able to walk afterwards. My sons were away . . . My husband went to stay with his mother for a week, and then went to [another town] for a job interview, even though he knew he wouldn't get the job, and he took his mother with him, and stayed for a couple of days for a break. He returned after I had gone to theatre for surgery. My friends, my old neighbours and the Christians at the Church, had given up on me at the time of my injury and first operation. I only had a handful of visits. I put this down to them being afraid that I would ask for help, both workwise and financial. I had a new neighbour who had moved in a few months before my accident and only knew her to say hello to! She has turned out to be good. The old neighbours just never came near except a couple of times, but again they were afraid I would ask for help. What hurt at the time was I had always helped them financially and with looking after their kids!

My own sons tried in their own way, but it was so difficult for them to accept I was now disabled in a wheelchair unable to do much for myself. They were so used to me being strong, physically, emotionally and mentally. Suddenly, here I was, just a little old lady in a wheelchair, unable even to shout at them! For a number of years that continued – they took over, doing as they wanted in my home and not even listening to me or my wishes. This was very hard for me, I kept telling them, 'I am physically disabled, not mentally disabled.' I also told them that I hated being disabled, and they didn't help me by behaving in the way they did. This annoyed them, and made them even harder towards me, but it did not change anything! After 6 years, I have at last managed to get my home back, and now I say what goes on in my home. I make the rules – sometimes they overstep the mark and break the rules, but I come back at them now, and each time I have to do that, I become stronger in myself.

Last, but very much not least, are my friends in ——, I had known them for a year before that awful day [of the accident]. They have turned out to be the only people I will ever trust, such good friends who have looked after me, and I believe brought me back to life. They care for me and others who have problems, but for them, I may well have given up. They have taken me to [their home], and got me well so many times over the last years. Yes some friends do care. I have lost friends, because they cannot 'hack' me being disabled, and don't know how to talk to me. They tend to talk over me; to the person who is with me! . . .

In the next narrative, Sarah conveys the psycho-emotional costs of living with ubiquitous cultural 'messages' about bodily beauty and goodness, about what is to be valued and what is to be despised. The knowledge that one will always fall far short of socially ascribed standards of beauty or acceptability can often result in negative self-image and poor self-esteem, at least until one finds the social and inner resources to assist in the assertion of self-worth.

Sarah, aged 50. She had polio at 1 year of age, leaving her with impairment in her lower limbs and spine. (Extracts from her letter.)

I guess I received many of the messages common to a girl brought up between the mid nineteen forties to early nineteen sixties about what a young woman should look like and be like . . . I was always invited to friends' parties. These were not very happy experiences. The emphasis was on appearance, dancing and the ability to attract a desirable male partner and the playing field certainly wasn't level for me. I had no disabled friends and few disabled acquaintances and tended to avoid 'them' like the plague. I still have some difficulty over this. Long ago I recognised that being close to other disabled people, especially those with similar impairments, was too like looking into a mirror. I have come a long way on this but expect it will be a life time's work to fully accept my appearance. Of course age adds complications and compensations to this. I know I'm not unattractive, I can dress well and look good but never to the standard I have in my mind. Part of this I think, is to do with the high priority given to physical good looks, dressing well and the importance of sport by my family and by the circle they mixed with when I was young. I know many people, I mean able-bodied people, suffer agonies they tell me when they try on new clothes or look at their perceived imperfections in the mirror. If I hear their complaints I want to say, and sometimes have, 'You think you've got problems'. I know about inner beauty, about beauty in the eye of the beholder, I even affirm now my own beauty. But if you ask about image, many disabled people feel the full negative weight of our society's notions of what is acceptable appearance which can wound very deeply. [Some] years ago I attended a self chosen, year long course on . . . assertiveness. At one point, two thirds of the way through the course, we were asked to draw how we saw ourselves naked, highlighting the bits we liked and the bits we didn't. For a long time I couldn't do it and sobbed and sobbed and tapped a depth of emotion and pain that had been bottled up a long time . . . Turning fifty almost exactly coincided with at last acknowledging that disability and I were inextricably linked. I have begun to work on some of my thoughts and emotions and to take an active part in changing people's attitudes towards disability.

Like Dorothy, Nancy's story is about rejection and abandonment by some friends and relatives, and her personal struggle to deal with and make sense of 'the hurt' caused by their inability to accept her impaired self. Part of the problem, in Nancy's mind, is the fact that her condition – arachnoiditis – is not well known or understood.

Nancy, aged 60. Nancy's impairment developed some years previously following hospital treatment for sciatica (a myelogram and surgery). She had returned to work as a sales assistant for a large retail chain, but soon experienced a rapid deterioration in her condition, experiencing extreme pain. A diagnosis of arachnoiditis was eventually made. In constant pain, she finds physical movement extremely difficult and uses a wheelchair. She felt that she could no longer work and gave up her job with a great deal of sadness and

reluctance. She lives with her husband who is heavily involved in providing
assistance. (Extracts from interview transcript.)

One of the most aggravating things to me is when your friends –
friends and colleagues – when you see them, say 'what is it, Nancy?'. I
mean it's eight years now and I think, well . . . if they just realize that
this condition exists, I don't want anything else, I just want them to
know it exists. You know I get really cross about that, as you can see. I
get wound up about that . . .

There's so many things about it, it affects all of you. It affects each
member of the family, sisters and brothers. My brother can't visit
without going away in tears, you know, and my sister can't handle it,
can't handle it. She's my younger sister by eight years and she can't
cope because I was always the one who did all the, you know, I was
the bossy one and she just can't cope with it really, so it's caused upset
there in a way. I used to find that hurtful and it's taken me years to
come round to the idea that we can't all do, we can't all care for the
disabled and, you know, we all have our limits, don't we? So the way
I look at it now – she has her own life and she's entitled to live it and
that's, you know, the best way I think, otherwise I was upset for a
long time. I expected her to be here all the time. You can't do that
really 'cos she's her own family also . . .

My sister couldn't ever deal with disability because her eldest son cares
for the very severely disabled people who have to be lifted and fed, and
years and years ago [he] brought one of the men he cares for home
unexpectedly and she went berserk. She didn't know how to . . . She
couldn't cope . . . She blamed her son for bringing him home. She said
he's no right to do that. Now this is while I was able-bodied you know,
and I suppose, in all fairness I've had to change, I've had to change . . .

I've friends . . . come maybe once a month, some every week, well
one every week . . .

I find the younger ones are more supportive of me. The young, fortyish
age group. They'll come and see me when they're on holiday, and
they've families of their own. And yet my peers, no. That's hurtful, that
was hurtful. But then, again you start telling yourself, well, they were
only colleagues, they were colleagues mostly, but when you spent
twenty years with them you know, you had a lot of things in common.

Fiona's account tells, first, of the psycho-emotional effects of living with
sexist disablism in the workplace, and second, of the damage to emotions and
self-esteem that come with being treated differently and insensitively by parents. Her narrative illustrates the close connections between one's inner state
and the way one is treated by non-disabled others.

Fiona, aged 33. Fiona has spina bifida, and now walks with the aid of crutches (she explained that she walked against the odds for someone with her condition). She had a very problematic relationship with her parents, especially her mother. She now lives with her partner. (Extracts from her long letter.)

I work [in] a male dominated environment. I do feel that I have had to be four times as good as the men to be accepted – I am a woman and also disabled. Once people get to know and work alongside me I am accepted and viewed highly by some people. I think that this has a lot to do with my hard work – again trying to prove to myself that I am OK and worthy of employment. Some people have a hard time with the fact that I am disabled, but also intelligent, holding an Oxford degree . . . If this is a real problem I just act dumb to keep the peace and smooth a few egos. I have had some trouble at work with sexual harassment. For some reason men seem to think it is OK to treat me like their young daughter – patting me on the head and putting their arm around me. Sometimes I wonder if they feel that they can try it on with me because I probably won't dare make a fuss (who would believe that a man would even have been interested in touching a disabled woman?) and maybe might even be grateful because I probably don't have much male attention in my private life . . .

. . . My father always blamed my mother for my disability and I imagine that it must have been tough for him to have a disabled girl as his first born instead of a healthy boy. After my paralysis at the age of 13 my father never touched me again, not even to help me cross the road. I still don't feel that he is as proud of me as he should be – or maybe he just can't bring himself to admit it. I know that he is very scared by me and what I represent and possibly what I have the potential to do. He finds it much easier to relate to my able-bodied sisters and is quite happy to hug them . . . My mother contributed [to my experience of abuse] by publicly making fun of my developing womanhood and passing very personal comments about very private parts of my body. As a result I always felt ashamed of any sexuality which I might have and removed it.

. . . My feelings about myself are getting better as I get older and manage to do the things that I want to. Long term therapy is also helping me to accept and look at those parts damaged in the past. My feelings about myself are closely linked to my physical condition. Five years ago my back suddenly deteriorated and after two more operations I ended up on crutches instead of being able to walk unaided. This really knocked me for six and made me realise that if I wanted to do something then I had to do it today because tomorrow

[it] may not be possible. My feelings about myself are also linked to feedback from other people. I need a lot of reassurance that I am valued/wanted/capable because I seem unable to generate these from within most of the time. On a good day I feel OK about being a functioning member of society – however it does not take much (e.g. being pointed and stared at) to make that feeling more shaky. As I have got older I have learnt to do the things I want to do anyhow and if other people have a problem with that, then tough e.g. going swimming in a public pool. But this takes a lot of inner strength and bluff and sometimes I wish I didn't have to keep fighting like this all the time just to do the things that others don't even have to think twice about.

. . . I still find it painful that whenever I go outside my house I am stared at by people and often treated in ways which would be considered totally unacceptable if done to an able-bodied person. All I want to do is to get on with my life but because I have a limp people assume that I am public property and somehow less of a person. Every person I meet will need careful handling – if someone is uncomfortable with my disability then I have to try and make them more comfortable. Turn the other cheek to people who are offensive as arguing back never seems to work. It just seems like such hard work to even just go shopping on a Saturday morning for a loaf of bread. If I am feeling a bit low then this effort can sometimes be too much and I resort to the freezer instead. I also wish that I could stop and explain to children (or adults) just why I walk the way I do so that they would not be frightened of me. Instead a child is hushed for pointing out (quite correctly) that I look strange and why I am the way I am remains a forbidden mystery to that child. I hate it when I inadvertently frighten children because of the way my body is. My experience with many able-bodied people is that I frighten them – I have to cope with physical problems and deterioration which they will probably not have to experience until at least 60 and this reminds them uncomfortably of their own mortality. I find that people generally prefer me to act the brave, uncomplaining disabled person who is always there to support them in times of trouble. I have very few friends who can cope with seeing me when I am scared and exhausted. Just why do I expend so much energy in pretending to be something that I am not just to keep the peace??

One of the reasons why I am particularly aware of the significance of the psycho-emotional consequences of disablism is that it helps me to make sense of my own experiences. As someone born without a left hand, my key experience of disability began as a child when I was made to feel by the wider society, but not by my family, that I had to conceal the fact that I had a missing hand. Being disabled is, in my case, more about the emotions and behaviours associated with 'hiding' the impairment for fear of adverse reaction if the 'hand' is visible in social interactions than it is about not being able to *do* things because external social barriers have been placed in my way. This is not to say that external social barriers restricting my activity have been absent (for example, I would have had an uphill struggle trying to enter certain jobs or professions because of reactions to my impairment, and certain teachers 'wrote me off' in my school days). But the motif of my experience of disability is the negative psycho-emotional aspects of concealment. I include a short extract from my own story here (from Thomas 1999).

Carol, aged 39 at the time of writing.

I was born without a left hand, an impairment which I began to conceal at some point in my childhood (probably around 9 or 10 years of age). This childhood concealment strategy has left a long legacy: I still struggle with the 'reveal or not to reveal' dilemma, and more often than not will hide my 'hand' and 'pass' as normal. But concealment carried, and continues to carry, considerable psychological and emotional costs and has real social consequences. This hiding strategy was partly bound up with school life, but looking back, I think a key influence was my association with the 'Roehampton Limb Fitting Centre'. Once a year from a very young age I was taken by my parents to this Hospital. My parents felt it was their duty to do this for my sake: to seek the advice of 'experts'. On these annual visits, my 'hand' was examined by a doctor who I remember as being very kind, and questions were asked about how I was 'managing'. As a result of these visits I was kitted out with a number of 'aides' like a strap which went around my left 'wrist' in which a fork could be inserted so that I could eat with 'two hands' like everyone else! The main 'prize' of these visits, however, were a series of artificial, or 'cosmetic' hands. These were ghastly, heavy and uncomfortable objects which I invariably relegated to the drawer soon after receipt. By the middle of my teenage years I had a gruesome collection of hands in the drawer. It was only some years later that I finally threw them away. I remember standing in front of a full-length mirror gazing at myself with the latest cosmetic hand on – how strange and unnatural it looked. Fortunately my parents never pressed me to wear these hands – leaving it up to me to make the decision. You could count the number of times I wore them on the fingers of one hand! However they did their work indirectly because the underlying message was clear. The experts were saying that my 'hand' was something to be hidden, disguised. I had to appear as 'normal' as possible. I found the easiest solution was to hide my 'hand' in a pocket, and I became very skilled at this concealment. Thereafter I always had to have clothes with a strategically placed pocket. So it was, and so it is.

Recent debates in Disability Studies: the cultural

It was stated earlier that the psycho-emotional dimensions of disablism are closely bound up with socio-cultural processes which generate negative attitudes about impairment and disability, and sustain prejudicial meanings, ideas, discourses, images and stereotypes. How can the origins and persistence of these negative social meanings be explained? These issues have been the subject of recent debate within Disability Studies and this section briefly reviews some of the literature. This links back to the issue of how to understand disability in social relational terms, discussed in the previous chapter. If disability is the social imposition of restrictions of activity on impaired people *and* the undermining of their psycho-emotional well-being, then to what extent can this be explained in purely cultural terms? Should we draw on theoretical perspectives which privilege the cultural, the discursive, or should we draw on those which emphasize the rootedness of cultural manifestations, and of ideology, in the social relations of production and reproduction in any society?

As noted in Chapter 1, one of the critiques of the social model of disability which has emerged within Disability Studies is the purported absence, or downplaying, of cultural processes in the work of leading social modellists, in favour of attention to material and socio-structural phenomena. For example, the disabled writer and activist, Tom Shakespeare (1997a: 218), has argued:

> Oliver devotes just two pages to the issue of cultural imagery in his major monograph on disability. Writers such as Finkelstein, and the prevailing orthodoxy of the 'social oppression' theories underpinning the political movement of disabled liberation are generally in accord with Oliver's position. Only recently have writers, predominantly feminists, reconceptualized disability. I would suggest that some of the lack of weight given to cultural imagery and difference stems from the neglect of impairment.

Shakespeare goes on to explore disablism with reference to the cultural meaning of impairment, drawing on research into the representation of impaired people in the media, in the arts, and in everyday discourse (acknowledging Hevey's, 1992, work). He highlights the typically negative images of people with impairments which prevail (freaks, objects of scorn and pity, curiosities, nasty and evil characters), and draws attention to the importance of Jenny Morris's writing on the nature of prejudice, especially her book *Pride Against Prejudice: Transforming Attitudes to Disability* (1991). Shakespeare reviews the usefulness of three 'theoretical models' for examining processes of cultural representation and objectification: 'ideology'; 'otherness'; and 'anomaly and liminality'. He characterizes the first model, ideology, as Marxian:

That is, ideas about disabled people are consequences of the material relations involving disabled people. Ideology is a system of theoretical domination, which justifies oppressive social relations. A determinist view, this privileges the material level of explanation, and does not give much explanatory space or autonomy to the realm of culture and meaning.

(Shakespeare 1997a: 224)

Shakespeare concludes that this ideology approach is inadequate, offering a 'mono-linear' explanation of the cultural representation of disabled people. In contrast, and drawing on Simone de Beauvoir's feminist analysis, he finds the 'otherness' model of considerable help.[5] In the same way that de Beauvoir suggests that women are subordinated to men through cultural processes which construct women as closer to nature, and thus 'Other' to men (that is, as 'Other' to the civilized norm), so people with impairments become 'Other' to non-disabled people:

disabled people could also be regarded as Other, by virtue of their connection to nature; their visibility as evidence of the constraining body; and their status as constant reminders of mortality. If original sin, through the transgression of Eve, is concretized in the flesh of women, then the flesh of disabled people has historically, and within Judaeo-Christian theology especially, represented divine punishment for ancestral transgression. Furthermore, non-disabled people define themselves as 'normal' in opposition to disabled people who are not.

(Shakespeare 1997a: 228)

The third model, 'anomaly and liminality', Shakespeare also finds to be of use, particularly the work on the prevalence of 'pollution' in ritual culture by the anthropologist, Mary Douglas. Here the focus is on the construction of cultural boundaries between those who are 'normal' and those who are anomalous, in the service of maintaining social order:

I suggest that any history of disability could be categorized along the lines by which Douglas suggests primitive peoples react to anomaly: by reducing ambiguity; by physically controlling it; by avoiding it; by labeling it dangerous; by adopting it in ritual. Historical experiences – such as the freakshow, the court jester, the asylum, the Nazi extermination, and so forth – can be conceptualized straightforwardly using such categories, and it is in this way that disability can be usefully regarded as anomalous, as ambiguous.

(Shakespeare 1997a: 231)

Shakespeare suggests that these models, particularly the latter two, assist us in understanding the 'psychoanalytical' and cultural processes involved in the disablism which result, among other things, in what I have called the psy-cho-emotional dimensions of disability. There is certainly evidence of these processes at work in the women's personal narratives presented earlier:

it is not our disability, but our impairment which frightens people. And it is not us, it is non-disabled people's embodiment which is the issue: disabled people remind non-disabled people of their own vulnerability.

The key features of this argument are firstly, the equation of certain groups with nature and the body, and secondly, the establishment of a normal identity through separation from the Other. Thirdly, and arising out of these developments, is the projection of negative attributes onto the Other, either as part of a denial of those elements in the self, or as part of a general denigration of disturbing, contradictory, anomalous or threatening phenomena . . . People project their fear of death, their unease at their physicality and mortality, onto disabled people, who represent all these difficult aspects of human existence.

(Shakespeare 1997a: 234–5)

Constructionism, idealism and materialism

The importance of Shakespeare's work in foregrounding cultural processes in disablism is widely acknowledged, although not uncritically, within Disability Studies. In his continuing search for theoretical perspectives of assistance, Shakespeare has also utilized Foucault's social philosophy, and recommends social constructionist perspectives more generally (see Shakespeare 1996a; 1997b; see also Hughes and Paterson 1997). Other Disability Studies writers who want to emphasize cultural processes have also been inspired by postmodernist and poststructuralist perspectives, especially the feminist disability writer, Mairian Corker (1993; 1996; 1998a; 1998b; Corker and French 1999).[6] In her work on deafness, Deaf culture, and disability, Corker argues against what she sees as the 'essentialist' materialism of the social model of disability. As a deaf woman engaged in a critical dialogue with both the disabled people's movement and the Deaf community,[7] Corker understands the social model to be based on a problematic dualism wherein the 'body' is separated from the 'mind', socio-economic structure is separated from culture, social structure is separated from human agency, and 'the social' is separated from the individual and her/his experiences. One result is that deaf people (and others) are marginalized or excluded because their oppression is mediated by phenomena which are sidelined in the social model, that is, language, discourse and communication:

> without the full integration of cultural processes into the model, reference to the cultural construction of disability and deafness seem somewhat hollow . . .
>
> . . . [W]hat is clear is that because human agency is lost in the materialism of the social model and because discourse is seen to be a side-effect of social structure, neither can be the focus for social change.
>
> (Corker 1998a: 38–9)

Social modellists of a materialist hue have not let these cultural critiques pass without comment. Colin Barnes (1996), for example, acknowledges that the Marxian tradition has undervalued the impact of Western culture in the oppression of disabled people, and states that Shakespeare's analysis, outlined above, is helpful. However:

> the main difficulty with his [Shakespeare's] analysis is that by endorsing Douglas' essentially phenomenological approach, he implies that all cultures respond to impairment in essentially negative terms. In other words, prejudice against people with impairments is, in one way or another, inevitable and universal. There are at least two problems with this perspective. First . . . there is ample anthropological evidence that all societies do not respond to impairment in exactly the same way (Albrecht 1992; Oliver 1990; Safilios-Rothschild 1970). Second, it reduces explanations for cultural phenomena such as perceptions of physical, sensory and intellectual difference to the level of thought processes, thus detracting attention away from economic and social considerations . . .
>
> (Barnes 1996: 49)

Barnes (1996; 1997b) sets out his own materialist analysis of the relationship between culture and the oppression of disabled people, arguing that 'disability or the oppression of disabled people can be traced back to the origins of Western society, and the material and cultural forces which created the myth of "bodily perfection" or the "able-bodied" ideal' (Barnes 1996: 43), and that this cultural oppression 'can be explained with reference to material and cultural forces rather than to metaphysical considerations and assumptions' (Barnes 1996: 57). Mike Oliver, too, has taken issue with Shakespeare's analysis, whilst at the same time acknowledging the importance of his insights: 'The emergence of post-modernism in respect of theorising disability is drawing attention to the important influence of cultural representation in shaping the experience of disability but, in Shakespeare's work, this appears to be reductionist [idealist]' (Oliver 1996c: 32). Oliver (1996c: 33) reasserts his own version of a materialist perspective:

> Hence the economy, through both the operation of the labour market and the social organisation of work, plays a key role in producing the category disability and in determining societal responses to disabled people. Further, the oppression that disabled people face is rooted in the economic and social structures of capitalism which themselves produce racism, sexism, homophobia, ageism and disablism.

In a helpful review of theoretical approaches in the study of disability, Mark Priestley (1998) has contrasted paradigms along the idealist–materialist and social–individual axes. Of those approaches which see disability as a social phenomenon, he compares the materialist 'social creationist models' associated with the work of Oliver and Barnes with the idealist 'social constructionist models' which are found in the work of those who, like Shakespeare and Corker, draw on postmodernism and poststructuralism. Priestley's analysis avoids falling into the trap of presenting one side or the other in over-simplistic terms, and attempts to highlight what is most positive in both approaches: 'I will argue here that this kind of oppression [disablism] needs to be considered as a product of both cultural values and material relations of power (such as political economy, patriarchy or imperialism)' (Priestley 1998: 86). In the final analysis, though, he finds the idealist approaches of post-modernist social constructionists lacking in explanatory power. He suggests that whilst these are very helpful in uncovering and describing the cultural and ideological processes and dynamics which constitute disablism, they 'do not necessarily account for *why* it occurs in particular historical contexts' (Priestley 1998: 87). I agree with Priestley's assessment that materialist approaches do have the potential to offer such explanations, and that, ulti-mately, 'the mode of production has a determinant influence on cultural values and representations and not the reverse' (Priestley 1998: 88). I will return to these debates, especially in Chapters 6 and 7, but now want to con-clude by returning to definitional approaches and the psycho-emotional con-sequences of disablism.

Endings

This chapter has introduced the argument that a social relational definition of disability demands that we find room for the psychological and emotional consequences of living with the daily manifestations of negative social mean-ings about disability and impairment. The psycho-emotional effects of dis-ablism are just as much a part of disability as are 'restrictions of activity' in domains such as employment, housing, and independent living. Disability is about both 'barriers' to 'doing' and barriers to 'being'. Understanding these barriers – their genesis, manifestations, prevalence, endurance – requires theoretical perspectives which throw light on socio-economic and socio-cultural structures and processes. In the following chapter attention is turned to a related issue, the place of 'personal experience' in Disability Studies and disability politics.

It is now possible to conclude Part I of this book by outlining, in its simplest form, the definition of disability I prefer to use. I am certainly not proclaim-ing this to be a definitive definition of disability – but simply one that comes close to expressing the thinking in this book and elsewhere (Thomas 1997; 1998a; 1998b; 1999).

A social relational definition of disability

Disability is a form of social oppression involving the social imposition of restrictions of activity on people with impairments and the socially engendered undermining of their psycho-emotional well-being.

Notes

1 I am not claiming that the psycho-emotional aspects of disability have been completely ignored in Disability Studies. Indeed, the work of Jenny Morris (1991), Tom Shakespeare (1996a; 1996b; 1997a), and others, pays particular attention to these, and to matters of self-identity. My suggestion is that, in Disability Studies in general, the psycho-emotional dimensions of disability should not be seen simply as additive to the real business of disability (that is, the socio-structural barriers which impose restrictions of activity). This issue is closely bound up with debates about the place of 'personal experience' in Disability Studies, discussed in Chapter 4.

2 It is worth noting that there is some interesting recent work in the relatively new field of the 'sociology of the emotions' (see especially Williams 1998; Bendelow and Williams 1998), which may be of assistance in Disability Studies.

3 See, for example, the work of Gillian Bendelow and Simon Williams on the sociology of pain (Bendelow 1993; Bendelow and Williams 1995).

4 In their communications with me, it was quite common for disabled women to refer to times in their lives when they were very 'low' and had contemplated suicide or wished for their lives to end. Their narratives told of their 'fightback' – finding a way to 'come to terms' with their (changed) circumstances and with other people's behaviours towards them, forging and sustaining an ontological security, and perhaps even finding ways to celebrate their lives (see also Thomas 1999).

5 See Chapter 7 for further discussion about the idea of 'constitutive otherness'.

6 See also the work of Janet Price and her co-writers (Potts and Price 1995; Shildrick and Price 1996; Price and Shildrick 1998) discussed in Chapter 6.

7 Corker (1998a: 5–6) defines the Deaf community (as opposed to deaf people) as 'that group of deaf people who define themselves or are defined by others as having a minority group status based on their linguistic and cultural difference, and who distance themselves from notions of deafness as hearing impairment and disability'.

PART II

FEMALE FORMS

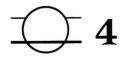 **4**

Disability and feminist perspectives: the personal and the political

Introduction

Preceding chapters have referred several times to the alleged exclusion within Disability Studies of the 'personal experience' of living with disability and impairment. Jenny Morris (1993a: 68) has put it as follows:

> they [some male advocates of the social model of disability] have been making the personal political in the sense that they have insisted that what appears to be an individual experience of disability is in fact socially constructed. However, we also need to hang on to the other sense of making the personal political and that is owning, taking control of, and representation of the personal experience of disability – including the negative parts of the experience.
>
> Unfortunately, in our attempts to challenge the medical and the 'personal tragedy' models of disability, we have sometimes tended to deny the personal experience of disability . . .

In Chapter 1, it was noted that one of the reasons for the apparent tension within the disabled people's movement along the gender axis was the desire of some women activists to emphasize the 'what it feels like' issues, and to make this the starting point for disability politics in opposition to male activists who wanted focus on the socio-structural barriers 'out there' and to remain silent about or downplay personal experience for fear of giving sustenance to the medical (and lay) view that being 'disabled' is a personal tragedy. In Chapter 2, the feminist criticism within Disability Studies concerning the causes of disability was briefly discussed, and it was noted that writers such as Jenny Morris and Sally French have argued, from the perspective of personal experience, that impairment *does* cause some restrictions of activity. I suggested that this argument is bound up with the problematic extension of the UPIAS social relational approach to disability in the work of some social modellists, one consequence of which is that what I have termed impairment effects are denied or eclipsed. Chapter 3 introduced what I have called the psycho-emotional dimensions of disability, distinguishing these analytically from the psycho-emotional and psycho-somatic dimensions of impairment effects. It was suggested that this psycho-emotional dimension of disablism, something which by definition cannot be understood without accessing and highlighting 'personal experience', should not be thought of as a 'private trouble', but rather as part and parcel of disability itself, and thus should be recognized to be of significance in Disability Studies and the disabled people's movement.

This chapter explores the theme of the personal and the political in more depth, drawing on feminist perspectives. This will help to unlock some of the reasons why aspects of disability, particularly the psycho-emotional dimensions of disability, have been overlooked by many in Disability Studies. In doing this, matters of epistemology come to the fore. First, though, it is unfortunately necessary to acknowledge the absence of disabled women's experiences, and of disability as a topic, in the work of most non-disabled feminists.

Excluded by our sisters

A number of women writers who are either part of, or closely aligned with, the disabled people's movement have spoken about their belief in the importance of feminist ideas for disability theory and politics but noted, with profound disappointment, that non-disabled feminists have failed to address the concerns of disabled women, sometimes actively excluding them from participation in feminist events. In the United States, for example, the socialist feminist authors, Michelle Fine and Adrienne Asch, who edited a path-breaking book on women and disability, put it as follows:

> Women with disabilities traditionally have been ignored not only by those concerned about disability but also by those examining women's experiences. Even the feminist scholars to whom we owe great intellectual and political debts have perpetuated this neglect. The popular view of women with disabilities has been one mixed with repugnance. Perceiving disabled women as childlike, helpless, and victimized, non-disabled feminists have severed them from the sisterhood in an effort to advance more powerful, competent, and appealing female icons. As one feminist academic said to the non-disabled co-author of this essay: 'Why study women with disabilities? They reinforce traditional stereotypes of women being dependent, passive and needy'.
>
> (Fine and Asch 1988: 3–4)

In Britain, Jenny Morris (1991; 1992a; 1992b; 1993a; 1993b; 1995; 1996) has argued in feminist academic journals and other publications that non-disabled feminists have sorely neglected disabled women, and that a combined feminist and disability rights perspective is necessary: 'Although we feel betrayed and excluded by feminist analysis and activism, many disabled women still feel that key aspects of feminism have great relevance to show how we experience oppression and discrimination' (Morris 1996: 5). For disability analysts such as Jenny Morris in the UK and Susan Wendell (1989; 1996) in Canada, the disappointment is the more profound because their biographies (shared with us in their writings), are bound up with the feminist movement: they were feminist thinkers and activists before they acquired their impairments, but as disabled women found themselves and their experi-. ences marginalized by their non-disabled sisters and from feminist scholarship.

Morris has advanced a particularly powerful critique of the feminist debate about 'community care', arguing that in expressing a concern exclusively for female informal carers in the wake of the excess burden of care imposed by governments' community care policies, non-disabled feminists such as Janet Finch and Dulcie Groves (Finch and Groves 1983; Finch 1990) failed to identify either with disabled or older women who received care, or with those who both *gave* and received it, presenting them as 'Other'. Thus Finch, Groves and other feminists did not challenge social stereotypes which portrayed disabled women as dependent, and so reinforced disablist ideas (Morris 1991; 1993a; 1995; see also Keith 1992; and Graham 1991).[1] Morris has also strongly objected to the tendency on the part of the few non-disabled feminists who have turned their attention to disabled women to pursue a 'double disadvantage' or 'double oppression' position: being oppressed as a woman on top of being oppressed as a disabled person:

> I always feel uncomfortable reading about our lives and concerns when they are presented in these terms. When Susan Lonsdale writes, 'For women, the status of "disabled" compounds their status of being "female" to create a unique kind of oppression' (Lonsdale 1990: 82), I feel burdened up by disadvantage. When Margaret Lloyd states that the issue for disabled women is 'the dilemma of identity for an individual experiencing multiple disadvantage and oppression' (Lloyd 1992: 208), I feel a victim . . . such writings do not empower me.
>
> We have to find a way of making our experiences visible, sharing them with each other and with non-disabled people, in a way that – while drawing attention to the difficulties in our lives – does not undermine our wish to assert our self-worth.
>
> (Morris 1996: 2)

Morris certainly does not deny that disabled women's lives are structured by the interaction of gender relations and disability – in fact this is central to her own analysis – but she is saying that in the hands of non-disabled writers the 'double oppression' perspective often serves to individualize disability because 'the attention shifts away from non-disabled people and social institutions as being the problem and onto disabled women as passive victims of oppression' (Morris 1992b: 89). Other disabled writers who have expressed criticism or disquiet about their absence from feminist thought in the British context include Nasa Begum (1992), Lois Keith (1992) and Janet Price (1996, see also Potts and Price 1995, Shildrick and Price 1996, Price and Shildrick 1998); in the US context, see also Hillyer (1993) – a feminist who writes as the mother of a disabled daughter.

There are some signs, albeit rather faint, of increased acknowledgement of disabled women by non-disabled feminists, and 'disability' is more likely to be included in the lists of 'differences' among women in feminist books and articles, along with those 'differences', especially concerning 'race' and sexuality, which have been a major focus for feminist debate in recent years. For example, Robin Tolmach-Lakoff (1989) reviewed some of the early texts produced by disabled women for a review essay in *Feminist Studies*, and the same journal later published a second review essay, by the 'disability scholar', Rosemary Garland-Thomson, which called for the development of 'feminist disability studies as a major subgenre within feminism' (Garland-Thomson 1994: 587).

Despite their disappointments with mainstream feminism, disabled feminists have got on with the task of applying feminist ideas in analysing disability, and, in particular, have attempted to make sense of their own and other disabled women's experiences. The fruits of their labours are of great significance for both disabled women and disabled men.[2] In the rest of this chapter I draw on some of the ideas and themes which are found in this work, paying particular attention to those which throw light on recent debates within Disability Studies and assist in the development of disability theory.

The significance of telling one's story and of 'writing the self'

The time has certainly come for disabled women to tell their stories.[3] In the last quarter of the twentieth century the years of silence (or rather, silencing) have been broken and the voices of disabled women are now in the public domain. I refer not only to the work of disabled women who are academics and researchers, which certainly include accounts of personal experiences (see especially, Hannaford 1985; Fine and Asch 1988; Morris 1991; 1996; Wendell 1996, Marris 1996; Corker 1998a), but also to the 'personal narratives' literature which has emerged in the 1980s and 1990s (see, for example, Matthews 1983; Browne *et al.* 1985; Deegan and Brooks 1985; Saxton and Howe 1987; Finger 1990; Driedger and Gray 1992; Mason 1992; Stewart *et al.* 1992; Keith 1994). These literatures 'give voice' to disabled women through scholarly writing, narrative and poetry – something that feminists identify as a key political act: making the personal political.

This 'bringing in of the personal', or 'writing the self', is a hallmark of feminist approaches more generally. The point to emphasize here is that the significance of this is not just that women's voices are heard for the first time – crucial though this is – but that it gives rise to new ways of understanding what knowledge is and how it is produced. This has repercussions for the development of disability theory because it reminds us that all knowledge is *situated*, that knowledge is a social product bearing the marks of time, place and social positionings. I would suggest that Disability Studies can learn a great deal of value from feminist insights on questions of epistemology, briefly reviewed here.

Challenging the status quo

In the 1970s and 1980s, many feminist writers invoked 'experience', both their own and other women's, as a way of getting women's voices heard and challenging mainstream (malestream) social science which insisted on a version of itself as 'objective' and 'neutral', as theorizing in a 'scientific' fashion at the level of the collective and the general (see, for example, Stanley and Wise 1983; Maynard and Purvis 1994). The purpose of giving authority to individual and collective experience was, in part, to expose these main-stream approaches as in fact highly gendered – privileging a male viewpoint dressed up in the scientificity of 'objective knowledge'. The view advanced by many feminists now is that knowledge, or ways of knowing, is *always* 'situ-ated' (Haraway 1991). As Bordo (1990: 137) has put it: 'There *is* no view from nowhere, indeed the "view from nowhere" may *itself* be a male construction of the possibilities for knowledge'. It was argued that the 'malestream' view of the world which dominated in the social sciences was based on a male sub-jectivity (the male subject as the 'norm'), and presented women, aspects of women's lives, and the feminine as the 'Other' (men as subject, women as object). The realm of 'the personal' was coded as female and was therefore devalued and excluded (see Stacey 1997). This, it was argued, was at the root of the shrouding from view of some areas of life as 'private' and therefore not of central concern to sociologists and other social scientists. By insisting on the study of women's experiences, feminists were doing two important things: first, bringing the study of aspects of women's lives centre-stage (her-story) and in so doing unsettling notions that some areas of life are 'private' or 'pre-social'; and second, challenging the epistemological foundations of the social sciences, especially the belief that there is such a thing as a scientific knowledge of the social which is unconnected to the social conditions (struc-tural, cultural, ideological) of its own production:

> Women's Studies in particular has opened up institutional spaces that explore the intersection of 'private' and 'public' discourses of knowledge, personal and theoretical modes of writing and individual and collective experiences; indeed, such dichotomies have themselves been under criti-cal scrutiny within such contexts.
>
> (Stacey 1997: 65)

For many feminists it follows from this that it is crucial to be reflexive,[4] and to 'write the self' into one's work – to tell the reader where the author is 'coming from' both experientially and intellectually, to make explicit the 'positionings' that inform the generation of new knowledge. Liz Stanley

(1990; 1996) refers to this as giving an account of one's 'intellectual auto-biography'. For some feminists, especially those who adopt poststructuralist perspectives, this 'writing the self' has become a major preoccupation, or been taken further – a full 'autobiographical turn' wherein new forms of writing are being produced which combine autobiographical and theoretical modes of writing (see, for example, Miller 1991; Probyn 1993).

> For many feminists the introduction of personal criticism [writing the self] is a strategic disruption of the smooth surface of abstract universal-ising theories that have constituted women in 'lack, invisibility, silence' (Miller, 1991: 7). The embarrassment that personal modes may introduce into academic settings touches on the sense that 'emotion', 'experience' and 'autobiography' have no place in the discourse of knowledge and should be kept outside the doors of the academy. The authority of theory relies upon the exclusion of the personal to maintain its status. For some, it is precisely these conventions, based in the traditions of objectivity and universal truth claims, that have been seen to protect the domain of Theory in the academy as a masculine preserve . . .
>
> (Stacey 1997: 64)

Disabled feminists

By taking the personal experiences of disabled women as their starting point and writing themselves into their own analyses, disabled feminist writers such as Jenny Morris and Susan Wendell are thus building upon well-established practices among feminist writers more generally. For the same reasons, in this book and elsewhere (Thomas 1998a; 1998b; 1999), I, too, write 'personally' and tell the reader something of my 'intellectual biography'. We are not dealing, then, simply with questions of stylistic preference, but with practices which flow from the recognition that knowledge is a social product, is situ-ated and positioned (Skeggs 1995a). This perspective on the social construc-tion of knowledge, and its corollary – the need to 'write the self' – has begun to penetrate malestream Disability Studies.

Some male writers in Disability Studies, most notably Tom Shakespeare, draw explicitly and centrally on the work of disabled and non-disabled femin-ists (see especially Shakespeare 1996a; 1996b; 1997a; 1997b; Shakespeare *et al.* 1996). Others, such as Mike Oliver, have taken some account of feminist calls for authors to outline their intellectual biography. Oliver (1996b) tells us something about his own 'personal journey' towards a socio-political under-standing of disability, and in reviewing the configuration of theoretical approaches in Disability Studies he also notes the importance of Jenny Morris's work in producing 'a feminist account of the experience of disability which was both a critique of earlier, male-dominated sociological accounts of disability as well as being a celebration of the lives of disabled women' (Oliver 1996c: 27). He goes on to underline the importance of developing a sociology of disability which takes the personal experience of disability seriously, noting that:

> My own initial work on the long-term effects of spinal cord injury [Oliver *et al.* 1988] . . . suggested that the occurrence of a disability [*sic*] as a significant event in an individual's life is only a starting point for understanding the practical and personal consequences of living with disability. The work further suggested that the social environment, material resources and – most importantly – the meanings which individuals attach to situations and events were the most important factors to be considered in developing an adequate conceptual model . . .
>
> (Oliver 1996c: 35)

Despite this, in recent debate between feminist writers and some prominent male figures in Disability Studies, including Oliver, there appears to be a major difference of opinion on the 'place' of the personal and the experiential – with the old denial of 'the personal' once again in evidence. I want to try to get to the bottom of these apparently contradictory trends. One catalyst in this recent debate was a paper by Liz Crow (1996; also found in Morris 1996).[5] Crow begins by talking about her personal debt to the social model of disability, and clearly stating that she is one of its proponents. However, she goes on to argue that 'when personal experience no longer matches current explanations, then it is time to question afresh' (Crow 1996: 56). What Crow then sets out is an argument for taking account of the personal experience *of impairment*: the social model should be renewed by finding a place for the experience of impairment. 'What we need is to find a way to integrate impairment into our whole experience and sense of ourselves for the sake of our own physical and emotional well-being, and, subsequently, for our individual and collective capacity to work against disability' (Crow 1996: 59). Morris (1996: 13) agrees:

> there was a concern amongst some disabled women that the way our experience was being politicised didn't leave much room for acknowledging our experience of our bodies; that too often there wasn't room for talking about the experience of impairment, that a lot of us feel pressurised into just focusing on disability, just focusing on social barriers. For many this feels a very dangerous thing to say, in that we feel it makes us vulnerable to non-disabled people turning round and saying – 'there you are then, we always new that your lives were awful because of illness or incapacity, we always knew what a tragedy it is.

These kinds of statements have been strongly criticized, in turn, by social modellists such as Oliver (1996a; 1996b), Finkelstein (1996) and Barnes. Before considering these counter-criticisms, it is very important to underline the point that this recent debate about 'the personal' has had as its focus the issue of impairment rather than disability: the terrain of the debate has shifted from the personal experience of disability to the personal experience of impairment. As I shall attempt to show, this is important because the impairment focus has served to muddle the issues about the place of the personal and the experiential. However, this very muddling has brought to the surface the persistence of a tendency among male social modellists to separate the personal from the social/political in such a way that key aspects of the personal remain firmly located in the domain of the 'private'.

The counter-critique

In his reply to Crow and Morris (and to others who argue in a similar vein), Oliver makes a number of points (for the full discussion see Oliver 1996a; 1996b). The one of most relevance here is that 'the social model is not an attempt to deal with the personal restrictions of impairment' (Oliver 1996a: 48). As discussed in Chapter 1, Oliver (1996a: 41–2) asserts that 'disability is wholly and exclusively social . . . disablement has nothing to do with the body'. He states that this is not the same as denying 'the reality of impairment' (Oliver 1996a: 42); it is not that 'the pain of impairment' is unacknowledged, rather that these impairment effects should not be the focus because the key political task is to tackle the social barriers which cause disability: 'pain, medication and ill-health properly belong within either the individual [medical] model of disability or the social model of impairment' (Oliver 1996a: 49).[6] Thus Oliver acknowledges the importance of impairment experiences but thinks that these should be dealt with through a social model of impairment, having nothing to do with the social model of disability. A second point is about political strategy: that attempts to integrate impairment into the social model of disability should be resisted because 'the collectivising of experiences of impairment is a much more difficult task than collectivising the experiences of disability' (Oliver 1996a: 51). Further: 'engaging in public criticism may not broaden and refine the social model; it may instead breathe new life in the individual model with all that means in terms of increasing medical and therapeutic interventions into areas of our lives where they do not belong' (Oliver 1996a: 52).

Vic Finkelstein's (1996) response to the arguments advanced by Crow and Morris is made in a less tolerant tone. Finkelstein objects to what he perceives to be a more general trend within the disabled people's movement and among Disability Studies academics towards a focus on 'experience':

> over a period of time, the political and cultural vision inspired by the new focus on dismantling the real disabling barriers 'out there' has been progressively eroded and turned inward into contemplative and abstract concerns about subjective experiences of the disabling world.
>
> (Finkelstein 1996: 34)

For him, the problem is that a focus on experience – either of impairment or disability – dangerously diverts attention away from the causes of oppressive social barriers. In fact, focusing on experience is a 'discredited and sterile approach to understanding and changing the world' (Finkelstein 1996: 34), leading to 'passive' pressure group politics limited to issues within the confines of personal experience. He calls for a return to a clear focus on the structural aspects of the social system, and to making common cause with other sections of the community who are oppressed by the social system (Finklestein 1996: 36).[7] I will deal with the points made by Oliver and Finkelstein in turn.

The place of the personal

On closer exploration, it becomes apparent that Oliver's position rests on the problematic conceptual dualism – the private and personal versus the public and political – which feminists have argued so convincingly against on epistemological as well as political grounds. His private/public dualism is well illustrated in the following passage, where he offers an example of what he calls 'the personal restrictions of impairment':

> As a wheelchair user when I go to parties I am more restricted than some other people from interacting with everyone else and what's more, it is difficult to see a solution – houses are usually crowded with people during parties and that makes circulation difficult for a wheelchair user. But other people may find circulation difficult as well but for other reasons; they may simply be shy. The point I am making here is that the social model is not an attempt to deal with *the personal restrictions of impairment* but the social barriers of disability as defined earlier by DPI and UPIAS.
>
> (Oliver 1996a: 48; emphasis added)

There is something very odd in not seeing this party-going example as precisely something to do with *disability*, or more accurately the interaction of disability and impairment effects. If we take the UPIAS definition of disability, cited by Oliver (1996a: 45) himself, 'the disadvantage or restriction of activity caused by a contemporary social organisation which takes no or little account of people who have physical impairments and thus excludes them from the mainstream of social activities', and apply it to his party example, we can see that Oliver is describing a social setting in which he is socially excluded (or disadvantaged) because the form of interaction between non-wheelchair users 'takes no or little account' of his situation and takes place in physical spaces (houses) which are not designed for people like him. Certainly he experiences impairment effects which restrict his activity by preventing him from standing or walking around, but in so far as a party involves social interaction in physical spaces designed by and for non-disabled people then disablism is also powerfully at play. Furthermore, it *is* possible to see how these 'social barriers' could be removed – if the party were held in a fully accessible location or space and if non-disabled people behaved differently.

What Oliver's party example really tells us is that, for him, personal experience is divided into the personal experience of coming up against 'social barriers' (such as being discriminated against in employment or in the housing market) and personal experiences which are 'private' because they are about 'personal life' and other aspects of the intimate. In this second category he actually includes *both* features of disability and features of impairment whilst referring to them in combination as 'the personal restrictions of impairment'. In particular, he collapses together what I have identified as the psycho-emotional dimensions of disability and the consequences of living with impairment effects. Personal experience is thus itself split into the 'public' and the 'private'. So, from Oliver's point of view, my application of the UPIAS definition of disability to his party example is completely inappropriate – parties are to do with 'personal' life, as are features of living with impairment, such as living with pain. Oliver (1996b) makes this double dichotomizing clear – that is, splitting the personal from the public/political, then splitting the personal into the private and the social. It is evident in the following statements: 'There is a danger in emphasising the personal *at the expense of* the political because most of the world still thinks of disability as an individual, intensely personal problem' (emphasis added), and 'there is a thin line between writing subjectively and exposing things which are and should remain private' (Oliver 1996b: 3).

It was this kind of private/public split which enabled some male-dominated left-wing political organizations in the 1970s to argue that issues such as domestic violence, sexual relationships and women's roles as housewives and mothers were not 'real' political issues because they were about 'private' life and belonged to the domestic domain (Rowbotham 1972; Coote and Campbell 1982). In Disability Studies, such a distinction sustains the view that some 'personal' issues to do with living with either disability or impairment effects are 'private' matters which should not be foregrounded by the disability movement. In the light of feminist critiques, this kind of dualistic thinking, this separation, cannot be supported. In particular, it was argued in Chapter 3 that it is important to acknowledge fully what I have termed the personally felt psycho-emotional dimensions of disability. By not applying his social model perspective to some areas of the 'personal', Oliver and others who adopt this position either miss out, or further deny, the *social* causes of oppression which operate in areas of life which involve self-identity, the intimate, the emotional, the so-called 'private'. This has the rather ironic consequence of leaving aspects of social life and social oppression which are so keenly felt by many disabled people (to do with self-esteem, interpersonal relationships, sexuality, family life and so on) 'open season' to psychologists and others who would not hesitate to apply the individualistic/personal tragedy model to these issues. Finally, the collapse of experiences of impairment effects together with aspects of disability into the same category of issues which do not belong to the social model, and are not of political importance because the 'real' issues are socio-structural, is singularly unhelpful to those who want to further develop a theoretical understanding of disability which is concerned with both the macro and the micro, with both structure and individual agency, with the socio-economic, the socio-cultural and the intimate.

However, whilst Oliver collapses together the 'personal' aspects of disability and the personally felt consequences of living with impairment effects, relegating both to a 'social model of impairment', there is also a difficulty with the way that Crow and Morris limit their discussion of 'personal experience', *in this debate*, to the experience of living with impairment and impairment effects. It is almost as if, in connection with recent discussion about the 'limits' of the social model, the domain of 'the personal' is always about illness and impairment. This means that Oliver can present his objection as being about 'bringing in impairment' when in fact it is a much deeper objection to dealing with . the 'private' or the 'personal' *per se*. The result of these two problems combined – that is, Oliver's position on the place of the private as outwith disability, and Morris's and Crow's identification of the personal with impairment – is that the psycho-emotional experiences of disability in particular get pushed out. In this debate, at least, they are not on anyone's agenda.

In her other writings, Morris clearly discusses personal experiences of living with disability rather than, or as well as, living with impairment *per se* (Morris 1989; 1991). But, as is demonstrated in the following quotation, Crow seems to conflate 'personal experience' with impairment experiences: 'External disabling barriers may create social and economic disadvantage but our subjective experience of our bodies is also an integral part of our everyday reality' (Crow 1996: 59). Perhaps the problem is that in arguing that personal experience should be brought into disability discourse and politics, feminist writers such as Morris and Crow have tended to go along with the 'restrictions of activity' definition of disability, that is, with what in Chapter 2 I have called the property version of the social model, and so have couched their arguments about bringing in the personal too narrowly.

The epistemological importance of 'experience'

Vic Finkelstein has argued that the growing preoccupation with 'experience' (of either disability or impairment) in the disabled people's movement is a dangerous and backward step. He appears to believe that 'experience' *per se* is about the 'private' domain of life rather than a 'public' domain of political struggle for disability rights. He asserts, as already pointed out, that a focus on personal experience is a 'discredited and sterile approach to understanding and changing the world' (Finkelstein 1996: 34). It follows from all that has been said above that I, along with most feminist writers, would disagree fundamentally with this assertion.[8] Apart from anything else, this anti-experiential position ignores the tremendous social and political gains made by a movement – the women's movement – which placed 'personal experience' at the very heart of its theoretical concerns and political actions. However, the issues deserve further consideration.

First, though, I want to make the discussion more concrete by bringing in some real life experience. Here is an extract from Nicole's narrative which, like the others used in the book, is a powerful demonstration of the way in which experiential accounts can act as windows on the social.

Nicole, aged 46. (Extracts from her letters.)

I hope to describe, how while needing intensive physical care, and assistance to live the life I want, I have learnt to be independent and have control mentally over all aspects of my life. Born with Cerebral Palsy, I am severely disabled . . . As part of my Cerebral Palsy condition I have no verbal speech. To overcome this difficulty I use a word board to communicate with people. This board usually sits on a tray in front of me which is attached to my wheelchair, and is approximately twelve inches square . . . After forty-six years of not being able to communicate verbally, one would assume I had become reconciled to this particular disability. To a certain extent I have learnt to cope in life without speech, and sixty percent of the time it does not bother me at all. However, there are still times when I find it both irksome and frustrating not to be able to speak verbally . . .

I was fortunate to have parents who brought me up absolutely as normal, encouraging me to think for myself and giving me opportunities to experience life to the full. Apart from six years at boarding school I lived at home nearly thirty six years. During this time I used to go into Homes for people with disabilities to give my parents breaks from caring for me. I didn't enjoy the times in these Homes, as they were run on institutional lines. I observed everything was done to a strict routine, and at the convenience of the staff. Residents were helped to get up in the morning at a certain time. Meals were eaten in a large communal dining room, residents requiring assistance in going to the toilet could only go at certain times in the day, and woe betide you if you were caught short, and all residents had to be in bed by a specific time. After one of these breaks I came back to my family home depressed. The reason for this was I thought I had glimpsed the inevitable life I would lead in a Home when my parents could no longer look after me. This didn't enthrall me, and I used to beg my parents to allow me to enter a Home just to get the dreaded business over with. However, my parents didn't listen to my pleas, and I am mighty glad, as the future has turned out very different from the one I imagined.

Twelve years ago my parents and I started to give serious consideration to where I would live in the future. I will always be grateful to my parents for encouraging me to leave home before it was absolutely necessary, while they still had their good health to be able to give me support in my new environment. I was very fortunate at this time as there was a newly opened hostel for people with disabilities in ——, three miles from my home. I applied for a place in the hostel, and was lucky enough to be accepted. Here the philosophy behind the running of the hostel was unusual in that the residents were in control of their lives mentally, but used the staff as facilitators to carry out physical tasks in everyday living.

With the staff as facilitators, I was responsible for every aspect of my lifestyle and welfare. I had to decide for myself what time I would like help in getting up in the morning, what time I would like meals, what food to eat, and be there in the kitchen directing a member of staff how to cook the food. In the hostel I had a bed-sit with a toilet attached, but shared a kitchen with four other residents. I had the responsibility to keep my bed-sit clean, and to this I had to book a member of staff's time to help me with the hoovering and dusting. In short nothing was done automatically for me, it was up to me to always ask for help I required.

I found living in the hostel both challenging and satisfying in that for the first time in my life I felt in control of my existence. The challenging part was remembering to do the little things that made things run smoothly, i.e. when I saw my medication getting low I had to remember to get a repeat prescription from my doctor, or remembering on a Thursday evening to get my money ready for the milkman. It was satisfying to be able to decide for myself how I wanted to live, for instance if I was having a busy day and only wanted an apple for lunch, nobody told me to eat properly. Similarly, it was satisfying to be able to entertain friends in my bed-sitter to coffee or even a meal that I had planned, directed a member of staff how to cook it, and had the meal served the way I wanted. I lived in the hostel for five years gaining experience of being independent. Then I heard of the Independent Living Fund which gives people with disabilities grants to employ their own care assistants. The idea of this concept interested me, and I decided to take independence a step further by living in my own home. Adjacent to the hostel are flats for those able to live more independently. These flats are owned by [the] council. Here again I was most fortunate in that a flat became vacant just when I thought of moving out of the hostel, and I was successful in getting a tenancy.

The next step was to find care assistants. For this I had the help of a care agency, who did the initial recruitment of care assistants. The agency then brought twelve women for me to interview and pick a team of four care assistants. While this was going on I enjoyed buying furniture for my flat, and getting things ready for the move. Then the big day came, and I don't think I have been so terrified. I was scared stiff wondering if this new adventure would work, and if it didn't would I have to eat humble pie and move back into the hostel? Would I get on with the care assistants I had selected, and if they would find me easy to work for?

However, this 'new adventure' did work, and has done for six and a half years. My carers and I have adopted the same philosophy as the hostel, i.e. carers are my 'arms and legs' for anything I require help with. This covers personal care, cooking, housework, writing letters to my dictation, planting my window boxes or driving me to visit friends, and places of interest, and much more. Due to circumstances, my team of carers has gone up to six. They work for me on regular days, and I have two care assistants per day. One works a morning/afternoon, and another one an evening. When I know I will be all-right on my own for a couple of hours, I send my carer home, but I still pay her for being on call in case of emergencies. At night I am on my own, but I have an emergency buzzer system to the hostel.

Once a month I pay my care assistants for their work. One of the coordinators from the agency helps me work out how much each carer has earned during the month. Then I go down to my building society, where my allocation of money from the Independent Living Fund is paid into, to get cheques. I lead a fairly busy life. Three days a week I attend a day centre for people with disabilities, where I do various activities. I am lucky enough to have a car which takes me sitting in my wheelchair, and this allows me to get out and about. I sit on various committees connected with disability. At home I keep myself occupied by reading, writing creatively, tapestry work, knitting and watching television.

The aspect I value most about having a home of my own is the privacy, and not having the pressure of communal living. Also its nice to have a pair of 'arms and legs' to myself, instead of negotiating with other residents in the hostel for staff to help me. It is satisfying to be able to manage my carers on a day to day basis. I always try to share out the tasks I need help with, so one carer doesn't feel over-worked. It's my philosophy that if I show consideration to my carers, they will give me a better service.

This detailed account of the day-to-day life of one individual, of her past and her present, tells us an enormous amount about disability and society in general: the importance of the attitudes and actions of parents and families, the limitations and effects of residential institutionalized living, the improvements in the quality of life which come with independent living, and the preconditions for a dignified and satisfying existence. In opposition to Finkelstein's view that a focus on individual lives and experiences fails to enable us to understand (and thus to challenge) the socio-structural, I would agree with those who see life history accounts such as Nicole's as evidence that 'the micro' is constitutive of 'the macro'. Experiential narratives offer a route in to understanding the socio-structural. As Elspeth Probyn (1993: 21)

has put it, 'experience itself speaks of the composition of the social formation'.[9] On condition that it is harnessed to a concern to understand the
material, ideological and discursive contexts in which life is lived out, the
study of experience (our own and that of others) is a very powerful way (and
sometimes the only way) to understand the world – a precondition for changing it. As Liz Stanley and Sue Wise (1990: 43–4) have put it:

> we insist on two positions. One is that 'individuals' do not exist except
> as socially located beings; thus social structures and categories can be
> 'recovered' by analysing the accounts of particular people in particular
> material circumstances. The other is that patterned social structural
> phenomena can be 'recovered' and analysed from the 'intellectual auto-
> biographies' of researchers . . . we categorically reject the depiction of this
> as methodological individualism, seeing this labeling as a failure to
> understand sociological fundamentals.

From a feminist perspective, Finkelstein's counter-position of personal experience to 'the social' is a classic expression of (malestream) scientism:

> Scientism has . . . been at the heart of the social science academic mode:
> grounded in Cartesian dualisms, in flight from the assumed nightmarish
> chaos of 'nature' and its relativisms and to the assumed securities of
> science and the foundationalism of its ways and means of knowing.
> (Stanley 1990: 11)

Finkelstein's unease with the experiential testifies to the deep-rootedness of
the private/public dichotomy and the embeddedness of an epistemology of scientism (albeit a social one in place of a biomedical one) in the dominant paradigm within the disability movement.

However, it would be wrong to give the impression that the category
'experience' has had a smooth ride within feminist debates. On the contrary,
feminist social and cultural theorists have debated the status of 'experience'
at considerable length in recent years, and there are now divergent views on
its significance (see, for example, Stanley and Wise 1983; 1993; Fuss 1989;
Stanley 1990; Probyn 1993; Maynard and Purvis 1994; Skeggs 1995a; 1997;
Stacey 1995; 1997). It is worth briefly reviewing the debates here because
they are of value to Disability Studies.

In earlier feminist writings, especially the emergent 'standpoint' writings
that 'gave voice' to women, and/or particular groups of women, the representation of experiences was largely seen as unproblematic: researchers
asked women about aspects of their lives and wrote it up. An overwhelming
authorial weight was given to the concept of experience (see Stanley and Wise
1983; Skeggs 1995b). In reaction to this, some feminist theorists criticized this
privileging of 'experience' (also characterizing it as empiricism) and tended
to argue for the development of feminist theory as if this was a completely
opposed activity. This, in turn, set up a 'theory versus experience' dichotomy
which standpoint feminists such as Stanley and Wise (1990) strongly rejected.
In reviewing some of these debates, Beverley Skeggs (1995b) states that

experience is always 'mediated': what we give researchers when they ask us to talk about our experience of X is an *account*, an *interpretation* or *representation* of our lives, and what researchers write up is further mediated by their own experience and their 'situated', and privileged, world-view. To say that these are representations or interpretations does not mean that they are 'fictions' (although some might adopt such a view). Rather, they are themselves the products of social processes which should also be the subject of enquiry.

Thus, there is not a straightforward relationship between experience, 'truth' and knowledge, and accessing experience as researchers does not mean that we access and reproduce something unmediated. The task becomes one of understanding the interpretations in operation (on the part of the researched and the researcher) as part and parcel of the substance of the experience related. Skeggs and others have therefore become interested in understanding how our subjectivities are constructed through experiences of living out 'discursive practices' – how we are 'gendered', 'raced' and 'classed' through cultural discourses (Probyn 1993; Stacey 1995; Skeggs 1997; see also Thomas 1998b; 1999). This 'be wary of experience as truth' view highlights the tremendous power invested in the researcher in conventional research: she has the potential to impose her own interpretation but at the same time can claim to be simply acting as a conduit for the expression of other women's experiences (Stacey 1995).

There is a strong parallel between this concern with the power of the researcher in feminist research, and recent debates in Disability Studies about the exploitation of disabled people by researchers, and the need for 'emancipatory research' (discussed in Chapter 8). The point to emphasize here is that the recognition of the danger of exploitative research has led feminist writers like Stacey (1995) and Skeggs (1995c) to underline the importance of making their own 'positionings' and 'situatedness' explicit – *writing themselves* into their work, giving an account of their intellectual biographies and interpretative frameworks, so that readers can more readily situate and contest their analyses.

Endings

This chapter has drawn on feminist analyses to unlock the reasons why aspects of disability, especially the psycho-emotional dimensions of disability, have been overlooked by many in Disability Studies. Feminists have argued that starting out from personal experience challenges conventional distinctions between the 'private' and the 'public/social' and thus both brings women's lives into the picture and unsettles malestream epistemes. It follows that feminists in Disability Studies have asserted that all facets of the personal experience of living with disability and impairment effects should be acknowledged, explored and made the subject of disability politics. We have seen that whilst having no difficulty with exploring *some* dimensions of the personal experience of disability, Oliver sets up a new division in the realm of the personal such that dimensions of disability in 'private life' get thrown together with the experiences of living with impairment effects and a new category is created: 'the personal restrictions of impairment'. Finkelstein, on the other hand, wants nothing to do with either the personal experience of disability or of impairment. He sees a focus on experience as a 'discredited and sterile approach to understanding and changing the world' (Finkelstein 1996: 34).

I have outlined my objections to Oliver's and Finkelstein's positions, but have also noted that Morris and Crow have tended in recent debates to conflate 'the personal' with 'the personal experiences of impairment', leaving the personal experiences of disability aside, and contributing to confusions about the personal and the political. This underlines the importance of making *analytical* distinctions between: the experiences of restrictions of activity, or limitations to social action, which are a result of disability (understood in its social relational sense); the experiences of the psycho-emotional consequences of disablism, or limitations to social being; and the experiences of living with impairment and impairment effects, which include both restrictions of activity and psycho-emotional consequences. All of these, singly and in interaction, should be the business of Disability Studies.

However, as noted in Chapter 3, from the point of view of the reality of lived experience, this necessary analytical distinction tends to dissolve. In the everyday lives of disabled people there is a melding of the accumulated consequences of coming up against social barriers which restrict what one can do, of having to deal with emotional and psychological consequences of other people's reactions to the way we look or behave, as well as the wider cultural representations of being impaired, and (for many) of the difficulties of living with pain, discomfort, fatigue, limited functioning and other impairment effects.

What would be the consequences if the feminist position that all knowledge is 'situated' were taken seriously in Disability Studies? At the very least it would mean acknowledging that all knowledge about disability (and not just the knowledge of the medical modellists) is profoundly related to the conditions of its own production. It would also require of all authors that they 'write themselves' into their work, at least in the sense of intellectual biography, so that the scaffolding on which their knowledge claims are built are made explicit (Skeggs 1995a: 24). As a result, apparent social scientific 'truths' about disability would be identified for what they are – 'situated' attempts to interpret social reality which can be contested and debated. In my view, all of these consequences would strengthen the development of disability theory. However, to situate myself, I should make it clear that I am not at all suggesting a slide into a postmodernist relativism (as some feminists have) wherein because all knowledge is seen as socially constructed it is believed that there is no 'reality', or no truths and errors pertaining to that reality. As a materialist, I assert that there is 'a reality' but agree that the way that we know it is always an interpretation. The best interpretations are those which can stand up to rigorous challenges from both empirical and theoretical directions.

Notes

1 I have to confess to being guilty of this myself in an earlier paper on the concept of 'care' (Thomas 1993). I was not aware of Morris's critique at the time of writing (being new to Disability Studies), and found it something of a revelation.

2 It is not just publications which need to be acknowledged, but also activity in the form of conferences, meetings, disability arts and other forms of cultural expression.

3 For an interesting discussion on the 'times' when oppressed and marginalized groups come to tell their story, see Plummer (1995).

4 To cite Liz Stanley (1993: 44): ' "Reflexivity" . . . [is] treating one's self as subject for intellectual inquiry, and it encapsulates the socialised, non-unitary and changing self posited in feminist social thought'.

5 Crow (1996: 55) explains that her paper had its origins in an article written for *Coalition* – one of the journals of the British disabled people's movement – which appeared four years previously.

6 We can see here that one of the threads in the debate is actually about whether or not impairment restricts activity and thus causes disability. This is ground which was covered in Chapter 2. The claim and counter-claim that impairment does/does not 'restrict activity', and thus does/does not play a role in creating disability, and is/is not part of the experience of disability are tied up with the 'definitional riddle' discussed there. I argued that the disagreements are to a large extent produced by the presence (and frequent conflation) in these debates of two versions of the social model position: a social relational conceptualization of disability (as in the UPIAS definition), and a 'social' variant of the ICIDH definition of disability in which disability is seen as a property – as 'restrictions of activity' of the person – which are then causally attributed to social barriers, and not to impairment/illness as in the ICIDH approach. The resulting clouding of 'disability as social' positions is no more helpful in the discussion between feminists writers and male disability authors within the disabled people's movement than it is in 'external' debates between Disability Studies writers and medical sociologists (see Chapter 8). As discussed, my suggested solution to the definitional riddle is to adopt an amended social relational conceptualization of disability. Then the 'debate' about whether impairment does or does not cause 'restrictions of activity' ceases to be a debate about whether or not impairment causes disability.

7 We learn from Barnes and Mercer (1996b) that Finkelstein's position has an early echo in the statements issued by UPIAS in the 1970s in its critique of the Disability Alliance which was dominated by non-disabled academics. For example:

> We reject also the whole idea of 'experts' and professionals holding forth on how we should accept our disabilities, or giving learned lectures about the 'psychology' of disablement. We already know what it feels like to be poor, isolated, segregated, done good to, stared at, and talked down to – far better than any able-bodied expert. We as a Union are not interested in descriptions of how awful it is to be disabled. What we are interested in, are ways of changing our conditions of life, and thus overcoming the disabilities which are imposed on top of our physical impairments by the way this society is organised to exclude us.
>
> (Barnes and Mercer 1996b: 8)

I can empathize with the disabled people who made this statement. Given the newness of radical disability politics at that time, I can appreciate fully their strong desire to shift the focus from 'what they say it feels like' to the external social barriers which disable. However, there is a world of difference between having our personal experiences written about by non-disabled 'experts' who see impairment and disability as tragedy, and writing and talking about our own experiences of disability and impairment. And it is now important to recognize, as many have, that studying and expressing personal experience is important for both epistemological and political reasons.

8 Finkelstein's position contrasts markedly with that of the American sociologist and disability activist, Irving K. Zola. In an appreciation of Zola's work, including his writings in Disability Studies, following his death in 1994, Gareth Williams highlighted Zola's view that writing about personal experiences could itself be a political act (see especially Zola 1991):

> Zola used autobiography and fiction not as an escape from politics but as a means of displaying the full impact of social and economic forces on the everyday lives of individuals; and, to paraphrase C. Wright Mills, Zola recognised that neither the life of a disabled individual nor the history of disabled people could be understood without understanding both.
>
> (Williams 1996b: 116)

9 I have tried to act upon this in my own disability research, for example, in analysing disabled women's accounts of their experiences of becoming mothers (Thomas 1997; 1998a; Thomas and Curtis 1997). I was interested in 'recovering', via the study of women's experiences, an understanding of the disabling character of the social structural and ideological features of maternity services, medicine and professional practices.

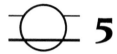 **5**

Disability and gender

Introduction

That the experiences of individuals tell us not simply about the *particular*, the micro-environments in which individuals live out their lives, but also about the *general*, the macro-environments which make up the broader social context of these lives, was an important theme in the previous chapter. As Mary Evans (1993: 8) has put it, when discussing the place of the auto/biographical in sociology, 'a study of the individual illustrates the social, and re-affirms the centrality of certain general themes in the lives of all particular individuals'. Or as Liz Stanley (1993: 45) has said on auto/biography:

> there is no need to individualise, to de-socialise, 'the individual', because from one person we can recover social processes and social structure, networks, social change and so forth, for people are located in a social and cultural environment which constructs and shapes not only *what* we see but also *how* we see it.

In this chapter I want to illustrate the tightly interwoven character of disability and gender by drawing again on accounts of individual experiences as relayed in the personal narratives of disabled women. I begin with a section largely made up of a series of extracts from the letters and self-recorded tapes received from disabled women, or from interview transcripts. These testify powerfully to the gendered nature of disabled lives. I then outline the theoretical challenge of understanding the intersection of disabilism and women's oppression.

Gendered disablism

It was noted in Chapter 1 that a growing body of literature on disabled women's experiences indicated that disability is always gendered. I suggested that the forms and impacts of disablism are invariably refracted in some way through the prism of gendered locations and gender relations, and that whether we are impaired and disabled or not, we all live out lives which are profoundly shaped by the social constructions of gender (even when we contest and transgress gender boundaries). I also noted that the personal accounts which disabled women have shared with me through their letters, self-recorded tapes and in interview cannot be made sense of without reference to gender norms in either their own or other women's lives. That is, whether or not their own lives followed conventional gender pathways (and most did), their narratives were constructed with explicit or implicit reference to public narratives (Somers 1994) about 'what it means to be a woman'. The majority of narratives are suffused with what we know from feminist research to be the 'normal stuff' of contemporary women's lives, with frequent mention of the following: becoming, being, or wanting to be a mother; being a single parent; being a grandmother; being a wife, having a male partner or boyfriend (sometimes in very happy relationships, sometimes not); good and bad sexual relationships with men; being patronized and belittled by some men, for example, by male doctors or men in the workplace; household labour and childcare; paid work and careers; women's health problems (other than the impairment(s) or illness in question); being an unpaid carer of others; managing the emotions of others in families and personal relationships (emotional labour); disadvantages in education and in paid work associated with being female; concerns about appearance, beauty, attractiveness; experiencing sexual abuse, harassment and domestic violence; matters of financial or material independence and dependence.[1]

Living with disability and impairment effects gives new twists to all of these. The list indicates that also running through the personal accounts are narratives which relate, not necessarily explicitly, to other 'differences' – of age, sexuality, class and 'race'. However, as noted in the Introduction, it is a matter of regret that the 'race' and ethnicity dimensions of these data are very limited: overwhelmingly, the narratives are bound up with being white, British and European.[2] In relation to sexuality, I was pleased that those narratives which dealt with this were not always about heterosexuality – there were accounts of being, or becoming, a lesbian or bisexual. One of my correspondents was a disabled woman who had had a sex change; of course, matters of 'sex', 'gender' and their interplay with disability are more complex in her case.

Choosing just a few extracts from the women's accounts to illustrate the gendered character of disability has been difficult – examples could have been taken from almost every letter or tape recording.[3] In making the selection, I have attempted to convey something of the wide range of gendered experiences by drawing on accounts by women of varying ages, impairments and social circumstances. Together, the narratives inform us very powerfully about the intersection of disability and gender, as well as about the significance of impairment effects, in the fabric of individual lives.

Sharon wrote about her life as an informal carer for elderly parents – a common role for non-disabled and disabled women alike, but one made more difficult because of the presence of impairments effects and disability. Sharon also touches on her experience of being sexually abused as a child, something which is now understood to be an alarmingly common experience of disabled children, especially girls (Kennedy 1996).

Sharon, in her late 40s. (Extracts from her letter.)

I was born with a very rare condition called Riegers Syndrome. I have very bad eyesight, [an affected] jaw, slightly narrower than normal throat, tinnitus, severe nystagmus which causes my head to nod at times and have a balance problem. I have a slight problem with my left side/left leg, a problem with both knees, a slight problem with my back and floppy fingers. The reason I haven't written before is that I care for my elderly parents. It takes me a long time to do things and I'm exhausted. The new Carers Act doesn't help me as I need some help but cannot get any. I sometimes drop things and can't carry heavy items. I'm also no good at getting up steps, e.g. to change a light bulb etc.

I'm quite determined (most of the time). I went to an ordinary grammar school and managed with great difficulty. I did office work for 15 years but haven't been able to work since 1980. I got the Duke of Edinburgh's Gold Award. I couldn't see well enough and didn't have any help to do an Open University foundation course. I would really have worked very hard to get a degree. I have a wonderful GP and he helps me all he can. Nurses and hospital staff aren't always understanding. I would rather not make any comment about my social worker, not in writing anyway.

I'm not considered 'independent' as I live with my parents and they own our home. I have taken responsibility for running it though (not financed). I've had 2 boyfriends (years ago), the first one was gay but I didn't know that at the start of being friends and the second packed me up when he realised just how bad my eyesight was! There were times when he was annoyed with me because I didn't do my share of the driving! I was physically, emotionally and sexually abused by my paternal grandfather. He did this torture for 12 years from 2 years until I was 14. I was not able to have children but if I had there was a 50 per cent chance that my baby would have been severely disabled . . . I miss having a reasonable salary. I always had a low paid office job. I don't think much of myself. Everyday I'm in pain, I feel unwell and am very, very tired . . .

Like many of the women who communicated with me, Sonia is a wife and mother. Her account of being a disabled mother is infused with the social expectations bound up with motherhood, and tells of the ways in which impairment and disability sometimes require the renegotiation of the sexual division of labour in the household.

Sonia, age not given but probably in her thirties. She is married with two young sons. She was diagnosed with myalgic encephalomyelitis (ME) three years ago, but has experienced symptoms over a five-year period. At the time of recording her tape, she had been very impaired for a long period, and had spent the last two years in bed, able to venture downstairs only a few times. She thinks, and fervently hopes, that she is in the early stages of recovery. (Extract from a self-recorded tape.)

When I talk to people who have ME but don't have children, obviously, they can rest a phenomenal amount more. I think one of the reasons I'm in bed such a long time is that no matter how poorly you are you've still got kids. I have to say I'm really, really thankful that I've got them because they bring life into the house. They bring their mates into the house. They bring all their, oh you know, ups and downs of family life which isn't restful but it certainly gives you things to think about, things to worry about, things to do, things that are outside of yourself. No matter how poorly you are, unless you're actually vomiting into a bucket, if somebody needs a note to say they can't do PE you're the one who's got to write it. Even if you can only scrawl two or three words on a page they still look to you to do that and I've really always done that all the way through, tried to do what I could, when I could, for the kids. Now, obviously I do physically far less for them. In fact I do nothing for them. They're becoming much more independent. They can sort and put away laundry and they can feed themselves in a basic way. They're probably more independent than most people's eight- and twelve-year-olds . . . There is one benefit to all us and that is, they know where I am [*chuckle*] 'cos I'm never anywhere else and they do get a fair amount of my time. Like in the morning [before school, the youngest boy] and I usually sit and chat or play cards or quadrangle or something like that if I'm well enough, so we get that time. My big one's twelve now . . . I'm always ready to talk, I'm always ready to listen except when I'm really poorly and I've got a bad head or I'm being sick or something like that. So I think they have benefited, they do benefit from the fact that I am always on tap. I think they've also benefited from a different sort of relationship with their father. We had probably a fairly traditional middle-class marriage. My husband went to work and earned money. I did a little job. He was pretty good round and about the house and he was quite good with his kids but he was very very busy at work. Well he's still got the same job, it's still as high-powered, although at the moment he is under the threat of redundancy . . . It's still a very high-powered job but he doesn't work at home much any more. He does what he absolutely has to at home but the rest of the time he's around for the kids as well. He takes them away on holiday. He's the one who takes them for new clothes and trainers. He takes them to the cinema. He's, he's a very good dad and I think they've all benefited from that change in relationship. They're getting a lot more out of their father . . .

Elizabeth's narrative describes how a relatively common experience among women in general – of developing breast cancer and receiving treatment – takes on other features bound up with being disabled.

Elizabeth, with cerebral palsy (age not given). She fought hard for her independence and cherishes her MA qualification obtained after many years of study at university (as a child she attended two 'special schools', leaving school at 15 after being told by the headteacher that she had fulfilled her academic potential). She lives in her own flat, but her elderly mother has recently moved in – as she put it, a case of 'role reversal'. (Extract from her long letter.)

I am extremely fortunate health wise, although having said that I have succumbed to the big C. This is an issue where I did feel my disability affected my treatment. My first mastectomy was when I was 'in care'. Complaints to the doctor about lumps in my breasts were dismissed as being neurotic! The unit's doctor was extremely condescending and patronizing – and very friendly with the unit's warden. I had a biopsy done, and was sent back for the result by myself. The verdict came as a shock, I had to have my breast off the next day. I was ushered into a cubicle and given a drink of water and left to absorb the shattering news alone, whilst the driver went back to the unit to find the warden's wife. The wait seemed an eternity! The warden's glib response to my state was, 'I can't leave you alone for a minute'! Up on the ward, I was expected to get into a bed with dirty sheets. My evening meal was plonked on the bed table out of my reach. I did not get a wash all week, other than when I was hauled from my bed into my wheelchair to do it for myself at the communal wash room. My dressings on my wound were perpetually soaked in blood because the nurses used to lift me in and out of bed by putting their hands under my armpits, this was excruciating painful because it pulled on my stitches. I didn't see a doctor once during that week until I discharged myself – still with stitches in, back to the unit, where at least I got more attention. Within two weeks of getting back to the unit, that puppet of a doctor declared me fit for work! Not through all that trauma was I offered counselling. After suffering in the hands of the NHS I decided to go private. My next mastectomy was a totally different affair in BUPA. Medical care was of the highest quality and all the staff seemed to be briefed in the needs of disabled people. However, the only criticism I have, is of the breast counselling nurse, who came in one day and said, 'oh well, you don't need me because you've been through it all before'. True, I had, but I'd have still liked to have talked it through with someone. It felt as though I had been dismissed and losing part of my femininity didn't matter. Maybe, my first experience of hospitalisation was just unfortunate, but I believe that when anyone is ill, they should receive the same standard of care, whether they are disabled or not!

In composing a fascinating account of her experiences, Faith decided to focus on the theme of care – both giving and receiving it . She was the mother of a young child when she became seriously impaired in the 1950s, and her narrative tells of her struggle to fulfil the duties of motherhood at a time when there was very little by way of social services or financial support for disabled people.

Faith, aged 67. (Extracts from two long letters.)

I caught polio in 1957, at the age of 27 and since that time I have been dependent on others for my care. I am 80 per cent disabled, affected in all four limbs, tummy and back. I cannot dress or undress myself, I cannot leave the house unaided and I am a wheelchair user. Over the 39 years I have seen a vast amount of change in the 'caring' scene . . . I was twenty seven years old and I had been happily married for six years with an only daughter of five when I caught polio . . . My one aim, at that time, was to fulfill my job in life, to be the same wife and mother that I would have been had I not had polio. No matter what the cost. I did, in fact, have quite a guilt complex, that through me, my family would have to bear such a burden, and it made me even more determined to make a home for them of very high standards. I was house bound, and found the isolation very hard to bear . . .

I decided that the amount of help a severely disabled person needs, particularly one trying to run a home, is absolutely enormous and that one cannot expect a normal family to cope with it. It is a permanent situation not a temporary one, which makes it much harder to deal with. I began to weigh up, very carefully, how much pressure each person could take and I try very hard not to overload anyone. I also try to accept graciously what each person wants to give me, although, quite frequently it may have very little to do with what I actually require, and whenever possible I try to spread the load. Nobody seems to mind doing a little, and you avoid all those horrible flare ups that happen as soon as any one person has too much to do.

. . . Because I spent so many hours lying down, I had a constant battle with my muscle power and it was a great struggle to keep it at a good enough level. Shopping was a major problem, and every day I wondered how I was going to get some food in to make a meal for my family. I felt that cooking was my forte and the least I could do was to have something ready for them so that they didn't have to start preparing dinner as soon as they came in. Eventually it was arranged that whoever was with me at lunch time helped me prepare something for the evening. One lady asked me why we couldn't just have beans on toast instead of making an elaborate meal. I said 'what, for ever?'

. . . In 1980 a miracle happened, my sister got married to a very caring man and from then on they helped me with the cost of some extra help. About this time, and as a direct result of the Snowdon Report another miracle happened. I was told that I was entitled to a home help to get me dressed every day and to give me four hours per week for shopping, cooking and whatever else was important. I found her to be a wonderful help and became extremely dependent on her. She actually took me shopping and I was able to choose exactly what I wanted, instead of having to look delighted and not show that what was bought was not what I wanted. The home help was also intended to provide some relief and backup for the living-in carer. It was extremely valuable both physically and psychologically . . .

Amy talked about her experiences of having a baby and becoming a mother. As a wheelchair user she encountered some prejudice among health-care professionals, although others were very supportive. I have written at length elsewhere about the issues surrounding childbirth and early mother-hood for disabled women (Thomas 1997; 1998a; Thomas and Curtis 1997).

Amy became disabled at the age of 15. The cause of her impairment is unclear – 'maybe a polio vaccine or a blood vessel in my spine'. The immediate result was paralysis from the neck down. She is now a wheelchair user who can walk a few yards with the aid of crutches. She did not give here age, but she has just had a baby and is probably in her late twenties or early thirties. (Extracts from a self-recorded tape.)

. . . No one that's a professional ever talked to me about sex, possibilities of motherhood, relationships etc. In fact, no one ever talked to me about any future. And this year I decided to try for a family and now have a five-month-old son. I'd a very supportive midwife but again it was up to me to find out what support was available. It's quite an isolating time trying to find someone with a similar disability who's gone through pregnancy and was able to care for a baby. Although there are organizations, it's very difficult to find people and to get together. I didn't really find anybody but in the end through reading books etc. I realized everybody's different and it's just up to you to get on with it. Most professionals were quite good during my pregnancy, except I came across one nurse who was appalled that I was pregnant and that I hadn't consulted anyone before I tried. I'm just wondering whether physically able women consult other agencies before they become pregnant? I've had support from friends but not so much support from the system. I've been through quite a lot of guilt in the early weeks of [my baby's] life that maybe they were right and I shouldn't have had a baby. I feel that I've got to be careful now not to over-compensate and not try to be perfect because of how I perceive, rightly or wrongly, the view that many people, and especially able-bodied women, have of other women with disabilities. . . .

. . . I think the pattern has been that society has a view of how they think disabled people should be and how I should act, but then when you try to break out of the stereotype you have to fight twice as hard. You've got to fight the stereotype of being disabled and the stereotype of being a woman and things that go against these two. Maybe the best thing is to stop competing with the physically able stereotype and just get on with it.

In the following narrative, Fiona (whom we encountered in Chapter 3) describes the experience of being sexually abused by a male doctor. Here, perhaps most clearly, gender and disability oppressions consort to produce misery and lasting psycho-emotional damage.

Fiona, aged 33. (Extract from her long letter.)

On the subject of sexual abuse, I am lucky that I have only experienced relatively low grade problems . . . The main problem I have had was with a doctor who I saw for about a year for pain problems . . . The first comment he made to me after examining me was 'well you can't be much fun in bed' as a response to the level of numbness/paraplegia I have. Then every time I went to see him, it was always out of clinic hours (I can't remember why). I would always have to strip off completely, even though I could never see just why this was necessary. However the doctor always knows best and so I went along with it. He would then examine my private area for what felt like ages and as I have no sensation there I don't know what he was doing – I always felt ashamed and dirty afterwards. I can remember that I became extremely nervous at every appointment, even to the extent where he once asked me if I wanted his secretary to come in if I was frightened he was going to rape me. I have had neurologists examine my private area to test nerve damage and they are always as quick as they can be and apologetic – this doctor was nothing like that. He was also not a neurologist and so should have had no interest in that area. After a year of these monthly appointments I went to visit him for the last time. I had to endure yet another long all over examination (I think that he also checked my breasts for lumps) followed by 30 minutes of painfully detailed questioning about my sex life, positions I used etc. I had gone to him about pain control, not sexual problems and this was the last straw. I answered his questions like a good girl (again my conditioning from earlier doctors) and left feeling physically violated – I have never worn the dress I had on that day, just in case I caused the whole sequence of events by wearing something inappropriate. Finally I made a verbal complaint to a female doctor who had referred me to him – she said that he would never do things like that and that I must have been mistaken. That really hurt – I know what my gut feelings had been at the time and I have only ever had them when around this particular doctor. Having my experience negated like this resulted in me pushing this whole set of incidents underground. It was only a couple of years ago when I mentioned it in passing in therapy that the true effect started to come to light. I still have to sort out what happened and how to cope with it. One result has been that I am very reluctant to see doctors (especially male) if a physical examination may be needed. This is particularly true of urologists and so I have continually cancelled my appointments because I cannot cope with the surge of feelings which come up whenever I have to be examined in that private area – for obvious reasons I cannot explain to the innocent male doctors why I am behaving so irrationally, so I just avoid even having to get into that situation. Some abusive treatment by a female continence advisor did not help at all several years ago.

Emily wrote about her frustrations in not being able to be 'a proper Granny'. This important gender role was difficult to fulfil because of the interplay of impairment effects (speech and mobility difficulties) and disability (especially others' attitudes, inaccessible houses).

Emily, aged 68. (Extracts from two letters.)

I am 68, and have had Motor Neurone Disease for 9 years. My legs and speech are badly affected, so I can neither walk, nor talk, properly. The disease has progressed slowly, so my husband and I have been able to adapt gradually as the disability worsened. At first I looked on the increasing immobility as a challenge – how to cope, and carry on doing the things I'd always done. But now I'm wheelchair-bound frustration has set in.

I long to do things on the spur of the moment – little things like change my shoes; pop out to the garden to pick some flowers; re-arrange the ornaments on the mantelpiece etc., [and] bigger things like, be a proper Granny, and help my daughter with her young family; visit Mother in her residential home; go on a shopping spree etc . . . Family and friends are very supportive, as are Social Services etc.; but I feel I'm losing control of my life, with most decisions being made for me.

I spend my time saying 'thank you' for services rendered – and feeling quite useless. The effect the disease has had on my speech is even more difficult to accept. The inability to communicate quickly and succinctly is extremely frustrating; and to see the lack of comprehension, and almost panic in other people can be devastating. I can almost hear them thinking – 'help, I can't understand her', or 'poor thing, she's brain damaged'. I can only use the phone to people I know; and need someone to speak for me when I go shopping . . . I would love to be able to be able to read to the Grandchildren – and how I miss a good chat! If I try to join in a conversation, I stop it dead in its track, as I usually have to repeat myself before I'm understood – by which time the thread is quite lost. Mechanical aids are a help with communication – e.g. answering a question; giving name and address etc. – but much too slow in conversation . . .

[Recently] I went to my daughter's for 2 nights to see their new home. They have a small bedroom downstairs with a cloakroom next door – perfect for Granny!?? The cloakroom is too small for the wheelchair, and with no grab-handles, sitting down and standing up was *very* tricky (as they are renting they can't fit handles). I managed, but went home with very sore tummy muscles! And all the equipment that came with me – wheelchair, walking frame, ramp, helping hand, etc. But it was worth it. What really got me was not being able to help with the children – getting them ready and taking them to school for example, reading to them at bedtime, exploring the country side, playing in the garden. Of course in the old days Grannies didn't do those things – but I don't feel old! Just useless and disappointed that I couldn't be more help. Our visit to my son was different in that we travel by rail, which we do a lot, and have no complaints. The man with the ramp is always there (well, nearly always!) and Paddington Station is well organised for disabled travellers. We use the 'Stationlink' bus in London (you can push the wheelchair on and off) when we can, or there are plenty of taxis that take w/chairs. My son lives in a bungalow with bathrooms large enough for a w/chair, and my daughter-in-law is a physiotherapist, so I'm well looked after there! . . .

With regard to 'care' – I am lucky in that [my husband] is my 'carer', and a pretty good one too. He has to do all the cooking and shopping and helps me get dressed – I can't put anything on, or over, my feet* – and helps me in and out of the bath. Once in, I can wash myself. Until recently we didn't have any outside help (other than equipment from Social Services, who have been very good), but we now have a girl once a week to clean the house. She is from a Care Agency who offer a wide range of care services. We may need to use some of them as my condition deteriorates – but it all looks very expensive. I don't want to dip too deep into my Disabled Living Allowance in case I need it for a 'Home'.

* I don't like having to be helped with pants and tights – especially by a man, even if he is my husband!

As in Fiona's account earlier, Gill's story highlights the gendered nature of disablism because it involves abuse by a man. In her case, though, the impaired status of the male in question indicates the complexity of the gender–disability interface.

Gill, aged 43, with Friedreich's ataxia. (Extract from her letter.)

My disability was gradually increasing and I was finding life more and more difficult. I left home (and took my son) and divorced my husband for unreasonable behaviour . . . I was unhappy in [that] marriage mainly because we were not suited but also because my ex-husband had a real problem with disability. This may sound crazy (as he was a paraplegic, with a broken back) because he was confined to a wheelchair but he could not come to terms with the fact that he was now a member of 'the disabled'. He would have nothing to do with other disabled people (I was the unfortunate exception) and insisted we live life without any aids or help. I found his attitude towards my disabled friends very hurtful and unkind. When I fell, he began hitting me because I could not get up. He would not let me ask for help and I eventually divorced him because I thought seeing me lying on the floor crying was doing my son no good at all, apart from the fact that my life to me seemed completely worthless.

This section concludes with two extracts from Monica's narrative. The first tells us about the intersection of limited expectations in education and the job market, bound up with being female and disabled.

Monica, in her late thirties. Monica is registered blind but has a small, though deteriorating, amount of sight. She was partially sighted as a child and was educated at residential schools for blind children, an experience of which she spoke in positive terms. Monica took part in a special school 'experiment' involving attendance at mainstream school for some of the time during her secondary school years. She participated in a very long interview covering many aspects of her life experiences. It is worthy of note that, at a later stage in her life, Monica was successful in re-entering higher education and qualifying in her chosen profession. (Extracts from the interview transcript.)

We had a careers officer come in to the [mainstream] school to give advice to fifth-years and we were given a seminar talk but also, if we wished, we could go and talk to the careers officer on our own, and this was actually suggested to me. I'd always had a thought that I would like to be in some sort of caring profession. I thought at the time that I would have liked to have been a nanny or at least somehow work with children. When I was about 15, 16, I actually used to go and help out a lot with the housemothers who were looking after the very little children in the special needs school and I absolutely loved that and so I suggested to this careers officer that I would like to go into some sort of career in caring, particularly for children, and quite blatantly I was told that that would be a waste of my time, because even if I got the qualifications nobody would want to employ me, so I was basically cajoled into accepting a further education course but in secretarial training. I went along with it then. You know, looking back now, I don't know why I did . . . [I was at a residential secretarial college for the blind until I was 19] . . .

... I took all my secretarial qualifications and got really good qualifications but when I started applying for jobs through the employment agency ... I was allocated a disabled person's adviser I think they were called then. They've changed the names now, but I was allocated this man who was a very nice man, I must say, who proceeded to try and find me employment, but nearly all of the jobs he found for me were working in typing pools which I had no intention of doing. I had got good secretarial qualifications and didn't want to work in a typing pool ...

... I was then offered the chance of going for an interview as a telephonist which, I mean, there's a standard joke between blind people that all blind people end up as telephonists, but that's what I did and I had no formal training whatsoever, I just went in, had the interview, got the job and had a morning's training from ... the Post Office that used to run the telephone systems ... I mean there were no prospects really with the job, but I must say I did enjoy the job because I enjoyed talking to people ... I really did enjoy that job for all the criticism from disabled people that blind people always end up as telephonists, I think it did me the world of good for building up my confidence but like I say it had no prospects at all. If I'd have stayed there, I would have remained a telephonist.

The second extract from Monica's narrative is concerned with the particular forms of isolation which come with being a disabled single parent in difficult financial circumstances.

I think the most negative thing I can think of is that I did feel very, very isolated. [My son] only being eighteen months, I didn't really seem to know anybody my own age or anybody else in a similar situation to myself because of my going to boarding school. I hadn't really made many friends in the area and those that I had made had seemed to have married people and moved on somewhere else and I did actually feel very isolated, felt very trapped. There were times when I felt very frustrated about the fact that I was bringing [my child] up on my own, and particularly when I was hearing stories of [my ex-husband] going out and living it up, and things like that. I suppose that applies to many single mums, but I really did feel very trapped. I mean I could take [him] in the pushchair and I could go locally, I could walk along the local streets and what have you, but I couldn't really just get on a bus and go somewhere I didn't know and take him for a walk on unfamiliar ground and just basically get away from it all, so from that point of view I did feel very very trapped and isolated from other mums. I never actually took him to a mother and toddler group either. When I look back on it now, I feel that perhaps I should have had more of a liaison with, I don't know, perhaps the health visitor or somebody like that, because my health visitor only visited me twice and seemed to think I was coping alright and left me to it, which I suppose I was, in practical terms, I was. In the house, I was coping OK but I never actually went out and met other mums until [he] started school, well nursery actually, at the age of three. Then I started meeting other mums, but most of those mums had husbands. I did meet one young woman who was a single parent and we did actually get on quite well and she seemed to have gone through a similar experience to me. Her husband had left her with no money . . . She didn't have any problems with my impairment. I didn't seem to be accepted very much by the majority of mums, but I don't honestly know whether that was due to my impairment or due to the fact that I hadn't grown up in their area because a lot of them seemed very cliquey. They'd all actually gone through school together and all the families were either related or had lived next door to each other for years and things like that so . . . I don't know whether it was directly to do with my impairment. I mean, I suppose you could say that the reason I went away was because of my impairment, but I don't know whether it was directly because they didn't want to talk to me because I'd got an impairment or whether they just didn't feel comfortable with me.

Making sense of oppressions

How can the intersection of gender and disablism be dealt with analytically? Is it a question of 'double oppression'? It was noted in Chapter 4 that the disabled feminist author, Jenny Morris, rejects the 'double disadvantage' or 'double oppression' stance which is usually adopted by non-disabled feminists (that is, the few who do address the issue) when discussing disabled women (Morris 1992b; 1993a; 1995; 1996). By doing this, Morris is not denying that disabled women's lives are profoundly shaped by both patriarchy and disablism. Her objection is to the accompanying presentation of disabled women as 'passive victims' of oppression:

> Images of disadvantage are such an important part of the experience of oppression that research which seeks to further the interests of 'the researched' must consistently challenge them. Therein lies the problems with examining the relationship between gender and disability, race and disability, in terms of 'double disadvantage'. Then research can itself be part of the images of disadvantage.
>
> (Morris 1993a: 63)

This point draws attention to the importance of *agency* in the extracts above: these women and the others who were in communication with me chose to tell their own stories in their own words, and their narratives are shot through not simply with evidence of 'how terrible it all is', but with accounts of how they survive, resist, transgress and 'fight' disablism and sexism – see also Thomas (1999).

In relation to 'race' and disability, Ossie Stuart (1993) and Ayesha Vernon (1997) have argued along parallel lines – that a 'double oppression' perspective which sees racism and disablism as simply additive is unhelpful. Drawing on the work of the black feminist writer, Carby (1982), Stuart argues in favour of the concept of 'simultaneous oppression', which suggests that the experience of disabled black and other minority ethnic people is made up of more than the sum of its parts (that is, more than racism plus disablism plus whatever other dimensions of social positioning are pertinent).

So, how should the intersection of disability and gender be theorized? One way forward might be to learn from feminist approaches to the theorization of 'difference', the subject of the following chapter. I want to close this chapter, though, with some observations on a difference of emphasis in this book as compared with some other accounts of disabled women's lives. The book edited by Michelle Fine and Adrienne Asch, *Women with Disabilities* (1988) will be used to make this comparison. As noted in Chapter 4, Fine and Asch's book was path-breaking in being one of the first to *analyse* disabled women's experiences. In their introductory chapter, these US-based authors reviewed the then limited range of published material on the subject and drew attention to the *differences* both between the lives of disabled and non-disabled women, and between the lives of disabled women and disabled men. In undertaking this important task, the authors tended, in my view, to overstress difference, constructing disabled women's lives as overwhelmingly at odds with gender norms. For example, when reviewing available data on marriage and sexual partnerships, they concluded that '[a]necdote, interview, and autobiography corroborate the census data and the stereotype of the disabled woman as alone' (Fine and Asch 1988: 14). Later they noted: 'We contend that men spurn disabled women as workers and partners because they fail to measure up on the grounds of appearance or of perceived abilities in physical and emotional caretaking' (Fine and Asch 1988: 19). This 'aloneness' also applied to disabled women seeking same-sex relationships: 'Disabled lesbians have described being dismissed, shunned, or relegated to the status of friend and confidante rather than lover, just as have heterosexual disabled women' (Fine and Asch 1988: 19). In relation to reproduction and motherhood, the emphasis was on the exclusion of disabled women from these experiences. On the other hand: 'Exemption or exclusion from voluntary sexuality and reproduction has not exempted disabled females from sexual abuse and victimisation. Perhaps even more than non-disabled women, disabled women confront serious psychological and social problems in ending abusive or exploitative relationships' (Fine and Asch 1988: 22).

Without wanting to reject the validity of Fine and Asch's observations, I have tended to put more emphasis on the 'sameness' or the 'shared features' of disabled and non-disabled women's lives. That is, whilst trying to illustrate the differences which disability and impairment bring into the lives of women, the effect of using women's personal narratives is to simultaneously draw attention to the 'ordinariness' of many of these women's lives. Thus, I have tried to illustrate difference in the context of sameness, so that disabled women are not 'othered'. To be sure, some of the women who corresponded with me did have lives which are particularly marked by being 'alone' and 'excluded from the feminine' in the Fine and Asch sense, but these were actually a small minority. Whilst there are certainly shades and degrees of this isolation and exclusion in all of the women's experiences, there is much in their narratives which speaks of 'ordinary lives'.[4] Perhaps my correspondents are very unrepresentative? In a strictly statistical sense this is, of course, true, and yet among them there is huge variation in the type of impairment, severity of impairment effects, forms and degrees of disablism experienced, as well as in age and social circumstance. Readers of books on disabled women's lives, and on disabled lives in general, will have to draw their own conclusions, but these differences of emphasis testify to the importance of a number of things: the dangers of over-generalization one way or another; the danger of constructing universalistic accounts of 'disabled women's lives'; the need to pay attention to the particular as well as the general; the need to give a nuanced account; and the need for more detailed empirical research which starts out from what disabled women say about their own lives.

Endings

If, as I have suggested several time in previous chapters, disability is rooted in the level of development of the productive forces, the social relations of production and reproduction, and the socio-cultural and ideological formations in society, then how does disability articulate with gender relations which are similarly rooted? Further, how should other dimensions of social division and difference be added into the equation: sexuality, class, age and so forth? The answers to these difficult questions are inevitably complex whatever one's theoretical perspective on gender relations, patriarchy, disablism, racism, ageism, homophobia and class, and I do not pretend to give finished answers in this book. However, some leads can be followed, starting with feminist debates about understanding 'difference' in the next chapter. Central to these debates are ideas about the 'socially constructed' as opposed to the 'essentialist' nature of socially significant 'differences'.

Notes

1 Of course, my 'invitation' press release listed 'areas of social life' that women might want to tell me about, including reference to 'issues to do with having or not having

children' and 'abuse – physical, emotional, sexual', and thus could be construed as inviting 'gendered accounts'. However, all of the items listed could just as well have been used, unaltered, in a press release directed at disabled men.

2 I am mindful here of recent work (Dyer 1997) which tells us of the importance of drawing attention to 'being white', that is, of not assuming whiteness to be the self-evident and unspoken norm which leads to addressing issues of 'race' and ethnicity only when 'black' and minority ethnic people are in the frame. See also Hill Collins (1990).

3 As discussed in Chapter 1, there is now quite a large literature documenting disabled women's life experiences which readers can also draw on (see the references given there).

4 I admire the writings of the American disabled scholar and activist, Irving Zola, and it is significant that he gave the following title to one of his books – *Ordinary Lives: Voices of Disease and Disability* (1982). See Gareth Williams's 'appreciation' of Zola's life and work (Williams 1996b).

6

Wherein lies the difference?

Introduction

In this chapter I want to examine the question of social 'difference' in some detail. Questioning and understanding difference has become central to feminist debates in the last fifteen years. What do these debates have to offer those engaged in Disability Studies? Feminist analyses of difference have not passed British Disability Studies by, and a number of authors have made it a focus of their attention, especially disabled feminists such as Jenny Morris (1991; 1993a; 1993b; 1995; 1996) and Mairian Corker (1998a; 1998b; Corker and French 1999), as well as Tom Shakespeare (1996a; 1996b; 1997a; 1997b; Shakespeare *et al.* 1996). In fact, as outlined in Chapter 1, issues of difference play a key role in recent critiques of the social model of disability within Disability Studies. Some critics have pointed out that the social model (or some of its leading proponents) has marginalized or excluded the experiences of particular groups of disabled people: women, gay men and lesbians, black and minority ethnic people, older people and children.[1] In addition, critics have argued that the interests of people who have particular forms of impairment are ill served or under-represented by the social model because their experiences or needs do not 'fit' the model – for example, people with learning difficulty (Corbett 1996; Warmsley 1997), deaf people (Corker 1993; 1998a), people with mental 'illness' (McNamara 1996). Interestingly, social class differences among disabled people are largely ignored, something which cannot be explained simply by assumptions that all disabled people are socio-economically disadvantaged. Then, of course, differences intersect: what shapes the experiences, for example, of black disabled older women?

Two types of challenge are raised, one theoretical and the other political. What are these differences, and how can they be understood and explained? What do these differences mean for individual and collective identity, and thus for political unity across groups? This chapter will examine some of the issues raised, beginning with a review of feminist debates on the nature of difference, then moving on to consider how differences among disabled people, and especially between disabled and non-disabled people, have been dealt with by selected feminist authors in Disability Studies. A discussion of identity then follows. The chapter closes with my own reflections on the issues covered, concentrating on what I see as the limits to the 'essentialist versus constructionist' parameters in debates about difference.

Feminisms

Grappling with 'difference' has played a key role in an increasing fragmentation of feminism into feminisms – but the new diversity is celebrated rather than lamented (Stanley and Wise 1990):

> Feminist research is now so firmly established that it has become diversified and (positively) fragmented. There may be fashions but there are no longer any hegemonies . . . we all no longer believe that we should write, do and think in unified ways.
>
> (Skeggs 1995b: 11)

Feminist fragmentation, theoretical and political, was the outcome of the application of its own logic of 'situated knowledge' to itself (discussed in Chapter 4). In the 1980s in particular, black feminists, then lesbian feminists, heavily criticized their white/heterosexual sisters for doing to them what it was argued malestream social science did to women as a whole: claiming to be representing the views of 'all' whilst, in fact, only representing the experiences and world-views of some (white, middle-class, heterosexual women). Those, it was claimed, who did not fall into the privileged categories were effectively silenced and excluded. As a result of the critiques by black and lesbian women, feminism became absorbed with theorizing 'difference' – both between women and men (critiquing as well as building on earlier feminist analyses) and, especially, between women. Feminists became increasingly careful to specify on whose behalf they were speaking and making claims – see Probyn's (1993) critique. As a result, much important work was done on the specific oppressions associated with sexuality and 'race' (see Skeggs 1995a). For many feminists who identified themselves as, for example, black, lesbian or queer, it followed that 'it is the exclusive prerogative of those who have experienced an oppression or a lifestyle to define its politics' (Stacey 1997: 62), that is, to claim to have greater and 'authentic' knowledge, or an epistemic advantage, in relation to being a black woman and so on. A number of feminist academics conceptualized this position as 'standpoint theory' (but cf. Stanley 1990; Hill Collins 1990; and Harding 1991). Thus, politically, the concern with difference manifested itself in a more particularistic identity politics, and quickly turned into the 'celebration of difference'. Supposedly 'despised' and stigmatized social attributes were reclaimed, owned and transformed into positively valued ones.

However, the recognition that the category 'women' is a falsely unifying one and that there is no universal female identity had the effect not of resolving but of dissipating the problem caused by 'unifying categories'. It became apparent to some that the construction of new categories – 'black women', 'lesbians', 'black lesbians' and so on – was not only a potentially infinite process (more and more 'differences' could be added on: class, age, specific ethnicities, and so on), but had the effect of setting up new universalisms, albeit on a smaller scale. As Margaret Somers (1994: 613) has put it, these new categories 'create a new shade of universalism that contains its own inevitable exclusions'.

There is another problem with the proliferation of categories of women based on differences, and with the identity politics which follows. This is the paradox that by identifying with and celebrating their 'difference' and division, women are reinforcing and sustaining distinctions which have been socially constructed within a male-dominated society. To put it crudely, was it not white men who dreamt up and are served by the maintenance of these differences in the first place: differences of gender, of 'race', and so on? Should women enthusiastically embrace all the categories constructed by the oppressor, and thus become complicit in the reification of these categories into 'fixed' types and essential differences? One of the founding features of second-wave feminism was its challenge to biological determinist ideas about gender. Is this undone by feminists who, in celebrating difference, appear to buy into the idea that there are essential differences between women and men, and among women? Arguments on these questions are ongoing.

Particularly in the wake of the rise of postmodernist perspectives more generally (see Chapter 7), the charge of 'essentialism' has been frequently made against those who 'uncritically embrace' categories of difference. It is worth considering essentialism in some detail here because, as I shall demonstrate below, it is of considerable significance in Disability Studies. Diana Fuss (1989: 2) defines the systems of thought which make up essentialism and constructionism, apparent opposites, as follows:

> Essentialism is classically defined as a belief in true essence – that which is most irreducible, unchanging and therefore constitutive of a given person or thing. This definition represents the traditional Aristotelian understanding of essence, the definition with the greatest amount of currency in the history of Western metaphysics. In feminist theory, essentialism articulates itself in a variety of ways and subtends a number of related assumptions. Most obviously, essentialism can be located in appeals to a pure or original femininity, a female essence, outside the boundaries of the social and thereby untainted (though perhaps repressed) by a patriarchal order.

In contrast, constructionism (or deconstructionism),

> articulated in opposition to essentialism and concerned with its philosophical refutation, insists that essence is itself a historical construction.

Constructionists take the refusal of essence as the inaugural moment of their own projects and proceed to demonstrate the way previously assumed self-evident kinds (like 'man' or 'woman') are in fact the effects of complicated discursive practices. Anti-essentialists are engaged in interrogating the intricate and interlacing processes which work together to produce all seemingly 'natural' or 'given' objects. What is at stake for a constructionist are systems of representations, social and material practices, laws of discourses, and ideological effects. In short, constructionists are concerned above all with the *production* and *organization* of differences, and they therefore reject the idea that any essential or natural givens precede the processes of social determination.

(Fuss 1989: 2–3)

Fuss notes that these positions are most clearly at odds when the question of the relation of the natural to the social is at issue: for example, are sex differences 'natural' or, like gender differences, are they socially constructed?

For the essentialist, the natural provides the raw material and determinative starting point for the practices and laws of the social. For example, sexual difference (the division into 'male' and 'female') is taken as prior to social differences which are mapped on to, *a posteriori*, the biological subject. For the constructionist, the natural is itself posited as a construction of the social. In this view, sexual difference is discursively produced, elaborated as an effect of the social rather than its *tabula rasa*, its prior object. Thus while the essentialist holds that the natural is repressed by the social, the constructionist maintains that the natural is produced by the social.

(Fuss 1989: 3)

For thoroughgoing anti-essentialists like Monique Wittig and Christine Delphy, for example, there is no such thing as a pre-social biological sex: 'women and men are social groups' (Delphy, cited in Fuss 1989: 51; see also Butler 1993).

Disability, impairment and difference

On the margins of these feminist debates about difference a few voices can be heard asking about the specific oppression of disabled women, for example in the work of Jenny Morris (1991; 1993a; 1993b; 1995; 1996) in Britain and Susan Wendell (1989; 1996) in Canada. What have these authors had to say on the question of difference? This section discusses, in turn, how both Wendell and Morris, while taking a 'disability as socially constructed' position, simultaneously adopt the view that there is an 'essential' underlying difference between disabled and non-disabled people associated with impairment. This is followed, in the next section, with a discussion of the work of feminist authors who adopt consistently anti-essentialist views on both disability and impairment. Together, the two sections provide an overview of essentialist and constructionist approaches which I hope will assist the reader who wants to pursue these matters in more detail.

Susan Wendell's philosophical reflections

Intimate as she is with feminist discussions on difference, Susan Wendell states early on in *The Rejected Body*:

> It should go without saying, but I want to emphasise that I do not speak for people with disabilities, or women with disabilities, or feminist philosophers with disabilities, or fifty-year-old Anglo-German-American-Canadian disabled feminist philosophers born in Brooklyn (well, maybe). In my opinion, no one speaks for anyone else unless s/he is explicitly authorized to do so by those being represented.
>
> (Wendell 1996: 6)

Whilst taking care to speak only for herself, and thus not to make claims on behalf of you or me, Wendell's analysis of the difference between non-disabled and disabled people, and of differences among disabled people, does draw lines of demarcation, and difference is a key theme in her book. Does she see these differences in an essentialist or anti-essentialist way? First, it is necessary to remember how Wendell defines disability and to keep this in mind when reading passages from her work below. As discussed in Chapter 2, Wendell's usage of the concept of disability is at variance with the British social modellist approach. She defines disability in the ICIDH sense to mean 'restrictions of activity' and, on this basis, argues that disability is the result of the interaction of biological and social factors (the social being the most important). Having discussed Wendell's version of 'the social construction of disability' in some detail earlier, I want to focus here on what, in addition to socially constructed differences arising from disablism, she thinks might differentiate disabled from non-disabled people. In other words, if the social oppression of disabled people were eliminated, would Wendell argue that a 'difference' between these corresponding groupings of individuals remains – a kind of 'residual' difference? If yes, wherein would that residual difference be located? To use Fuss's terms above, is it an *essential* difference – a pre-social, 'natural', 'real' biological difference?

On this point, there is an essentialist thread in Wendell's analysis. She talks about her 'emerging understanding of disability as socially constructed *from biological differences* between the disabled and the non-disabled' (Wendell 1996: 5; emphasis added), and refers in places to 'biological reality underlying distinctions' between disabled and non-disabled people. Wendell is certainly very well aware that the social meanings ('normal', 'abnormal') attached to these biological differences can and do vary within and between societies and over time, and she advances a sophisticated analysis of the contemporary cultural construction of disability, but nevertheless she appears to accept that there *are* biological differences which really do set some bodies apart from others, irrespective of the social labels that might or might not be attached to these 'differences'; socially constructed differences *overlie* essential bodily differences. Her position becomes clearest when she critiques non-disabled feminist's work on 'the body'. Heavily influenced by constructionist ideas, this mainstream feminist work on the body implies that there are no such things as 'real', material bodies. She says:

> I want to distinguish [my] view from approaches to cultural construction of 'the body' that seem to confuse the lived reality of bodies with cultural discourse about and representations of bodies, or that deny or ignore bodily experience in favour of fascination with bodily representations . . . I do not think my body is a cultural representation, although I recognise that my experience of it is both highly interpreted and very influenced by cultural (including medical) representations. Moreover, I think it would be cruel, as well as a distortion of people's lives, to erase or ignore the everyday, practical, experienced limitations of people's disabilities [restrictions of activity] simply because we recognise that human bodies and their varied conditions are both changeable and highly interpreted.
>
> (Wendell 1996: 44)

Wendell also considers whether or not the differences *among* disabled people work for or against the possibility of a common 'disabled' identity – a perception of commonality which is a necessary precondition for a disability politics and a disability culture – irrespective of any underlying essential sameness. As a feminist, she is not surprisingly at pains to emphasize diversity and to avoid masking 'difference':

> We now know, from the extensive writings of women with disabilities, that living with similar disabilities is different for females and males. An emerging literature also reveals that living with similar disabilities is different for women of different races, classes, sexual identities, and ethnicities.
>
> (Wendell 1996: 70)

Thus for any individual with impairment, their 'essential' difference is overlaid not only with the socially constructed differences associated with disability, but also with many other constructions associated with gender, 'race', sexuality and so on. However, despite these many differences between disabled people, Wendell (1996: 32) concludes:

> I think 'people with disabilities' is not a meaningless category as long as there is social oppression based on disability, even though the forms this oppression takes, and the ways it is experienced, may vary greatly among societies and according to other factors, such as age, gender, race, class, religion, caste, and sexual identity.

Wendell (1996: 69) raises the question of whether there can be a 'standpoint epistemology for people with disabilities': would this be falsely universalizing?

She carefully considers the arguments for and against this possibility, and tentatively concludes that disabled people do have an epistemic advantage:

> Does having a disability in itself give a person a particular point of view or a less distorted and complete perspective on certain issues? No. Following in the footsteps of Patricia Hill Collins, I want to say that having a disability usually gives a person experiences of the world different from people without disabilities, and that being a woman with a disability usually gives a person different experiences from those of people who are not female and disabled, and that these different experiences create the possibility of different perspectives which have epistemic advantages with respect to certain issues. I do not claim that all people with disabilities, or all women with disabilities, have the same epistemic advantages, or that they all have the same interpretations of their experiences, or even that they have similar experiences. We are just beginning to investigate how much we have in common . . . I do want to claim that, collectively, we have accumulated a significant body of knowledge, with a different standpoint (or standpoints) from those without disabilities, and that that knowledge, which has been ignored and repressed in non-disabled culture should be further developed and articulated.
>
> (Wendell 1996: 73)

This idea that 'people with disabilities have both knowledge and ways of knowing that are not available to the non-disabled' (Wendell 1996: 75) is an important one in Wendell's analysis. The features of this knowledge that are emphasized are: 'the knowledge that people with disabilities have about living with bodily suffering and limitation and about how their cultures treat rejected aspects of bodily life' (Wendell 1996: 5), and the knowledge that individuals might *gain* something from their experiences of living with disability and that some forms of bodily difference are to be valued (Wendell 1996: 66–7). Thus some of the differences are, or give rise to, valued and celebrated differences. Wendell (1996: 69) states that if such epistemic knowledge ceased to be socially discounted, and came to be acknowledged by non-disabled people, then 'it would enrich and expand our culture, and some of it has the potential to change our thinking and our ways of life profoundly'. Thus, for Wendell, difference between disabled and non-disabled people is both essential and socially constructed.

Jenny Morris on difference

As a feminist writer, Jenny Morris is also very sensitive to 'difference'. Much of her work attempts to bring the differences associated with disability to the attention of mainstream feminism on the one hand, and to bring gender differences among disabled people to the attention of Disability Studies and the disabled people's movement on the other (Morris 1991; 1993a; 1993b; 1995; 1996). I discussed Morris's assessment of the failure of non-disabled feminists to acknowledge disabled women in Chapter 4, so what does she say about the significance of gender differences in relation to disability scholarship and practice?

> Disability research and theory either treats gender as invisible or separates the issue out into a focus on the experiences of disabled women. Thus, research often assumes the experience of disabled men to be representative of the disabled experience in general, and, when gender is introduced into the discussion, it is commonly in terms of disabled women experiencing a 'double disadvantage'. However, if we give full recognition to the importance of gender, the experience of both disabled men and disabled women will be more closely represented and explained.
>
> (Morris 1993b: 85)

By either 'othering' disabled women, or claiming to speak for 'disabled people' when in fact it is the experience of disabled men that is articulated, Morris argues that most men within Disability Studies have effectively elided gender differences and ignored the gendered character of disability.[2] In her view the socially constructed natures of both disability and gender mean that the experience of disability is inevitably a gendered one, and thus a different one for men and women. It follows that Morris also acknowledges that the experience of disability is also 'raced', 'classed', 'aged' and so forth.

However, I would suggest that Morris tends not to push this analysis of difference among disabled people, and thus of who can speak for whom, far enough. For example, in much of her work she implicitly or explicitly speaks for 'disabled women' in a way which makes me rather uneasy; inevitably the differences among disabled women become obscured. This is particularly the case in *Pride Against Prejudice: Transforming Attitudes to Disability* (1991), but is also evident in her later edited volume, *Encounters with Strangers: Feminism and Disability* (1996), where she frequently claims to be talking on behalf of disabled women as a whole by making claims on behalf of 'us'. As in feminist identity politics in general, there is also a strong call to 'celebrate' the difference. For example:

> But we are different. We reject the meanings that the non-disabled world attaches to disability but we do not reject the differences which are such an important part of our identities.
>
> We can assert the importance of our experience for the whole of society, and insist on our rights to be integrated within our communities. However, it is important that we are explicit about the ways in which we are not like the non-disabled world. By claiming our own definitions of disability we can also take pride in our abnormality, our difference.
>
> (Morris 1991: 16–17)

Most of the people we have dealings with, including our most intimate relationships, are not like us. It is therefore very difficult for us to recognise and challenge the values and judgments that are applied to us and our lives. Our ideas about disability and about ourselves are generally formed by those who are not disabled.

(Morris 1991: 37)

We are outraged that our voices are silenced so that our oppression is not recognised; we define as injustice the exclusion of disabled people from mainstream society.

In doing this we share with each other, and develop an understanding of, the detailed reality of our lives, using such politicisation of the personal to make sense of our experiences of prejudice and discrimination.

(Morris 1996: 4)

Perhaps the political imperative of putting disabled women on the map, of making 'us' visible, outweighs the necessity of being cautious about speaking for others, assuming commonalties, and creating 'new shades of universalism'? In my view there is no doubt that Morris's work is of tremendous political significance for disabled women, but I would have expected her to qualify her use of 'we'. Perhaps I am particularly sensitive on this point because some of the things Morris says on my behalf (as a disabled woman), are not wholly true for me, and may not, therefore, be true for others. One example concerns the issue of 'passing' as normal, usually through disguising an impairment or by failing to bring a 'not obvious' impairment to the attention of others in social interactions. In *Pride Against Prejudice*, Morris argues that passing is a denial of what we 'really are'; it is to 'present ourselves as an exception to the category to which we otherwise belong' (Morris 1991: 37). As someone who often 'passes' as normal (as indicated in Chapter 3), sometimes through purposive concealment and sometimes because of the 'not always obvious' nature of my impairment in particular contexts, I have mixed feelings about Morris's claims. Her message is clear: by not bringing a disabled identity into the open on all occasions, my behaviour undermines the lives of, and thus betrays, other disabled people. Whilst I agree with this painful truth in some ways, it does not acknowledge either the particularities of my impairment and disability experiences, or the 'burden' that would be shouldered by continually having to make visible a not very visible difference. As a wheelchair user, Morris may not be confronted with the same sorts of dilemmas. Specifically, her argument may not represent the experiences of those disabled women who, like me, live in the borderlands between the disabled and non-disabled worlds because 'our' impairments are sometimes visible and sometimes not. In other words, Morris's analysis is not sufficiently nuanced; it sometimes assumes too much 'sameness' based on her own experiences.

In addition, if I were always to make a point of bringing my disabled status to people's attention, I would effectively be making my 'disabled identity' my dominant or 'master status' (Goffman 1963). But many feminists would say that identities are not singular but are multiple and 'fractured'. As well as being a disabled person, I am a woman, I am white, I am a mother, I am middle class . . . and many other things; all of these could be seen to be fragments of my identity, or as discursive constructions which constitute my identity. I will return to the issue of identity later in the chapter. What I want to emphasize here is that the impression given in Morris's writing is that being disabled is always the *key* difference between 'ourselves' and 'others'.

Moving on, what exactly does Morris mean when she asserts in the passage quoted above that 'we are different'? Is it an entirely socially constructed difference, or is there some underlying 'essential' difference in addition to 'being disabled' by social barriers? Like Wendell, Morris appears to begin from an essentialist premise that being impaired or chronically ill constitutes an essential (pre-social) difference, although she too acknowledges that these differences can carry different social meanings in different social and cultural contexts:

> we are often physically different from what is considered to be the norm, the average person . . . Our bodies generally look and behave differently from most other people's (even if we have an invisible physical [impairment] there is usually something about the way our bodies behave which gives our difference away). It is not normal to have difficulty walking or to be unable to walk; it is not normal to be unable to see, to hear; it is not normal to be incontinent, to have fits, to experience extreme tiredness, to be in constant pain; it is not normal to have a limb or limbs missing. If we have a learning disability the way we interact with others usually reveals our difference.
>
> These are the types of intellectual and physical characteristics which distinguish our experience from that of the majority of the population. They are all part of the human experience but they are not the norm; that is, most people at any one point in time do not experience them, although many may experience them.
>
> (Morris 1991: 17)

Thus Morris posits a distinction between the impaired (not normal) body and the unimpaired (normal) body which exists prior to social differences; using Fuss's language, social differences are mapped on to, *a posteriori*, the biological subject. This gives rise to experiences which are unique to living with impairment. Operating as the physical markers for social discrimination, impairments give rise, in turn, to unique experiences of social oppression. So, like Wendell, Morris suggests that there is an *essential* difference between impaired and non-impaired individuals *in addition to*, or as a substratum of, socially constructed differences consequent upon disablism in society and culture. And like Wendell, Morris draws attention to the valued nature of 'our differences': 'Physical disability and illness are an important part of human experience . . . and given the chance, can create important and different ways of looking at things' (Morris 1991: 38).

Constructed difference?

If one follows the lead of feminist anti-essentialists who deconstruct categories such as 'sex' and 'race', one has to consider the possibility that Wendell and

Morris might be trapped in the tramlines of modernist discourses and that the category of 'impairment', and the status of 'being impaired', are entirely socially constructed, that is, categories wholly constituted through discursive practices. A thoroughgoing deconstructionist approach would reject any notion that there is an 'essential' body which can be said to be the 'normal' body, and thus sets the criteria for the 'impaired' body. Anti-essentialists would look for the 'intricate and interlacing processes which work together to produce' (Fuss 1989: 2) the seemingly 'natural' or 'normal' body. These processes would consist of systems of representations, social and material practices, discourses, and ideological effects. The question becomes: how is the 'impaired' body produced and organized in society? And how are the 'impaired' body and the 'disabled' person also 'sexed', 'gendered', 'raced', and so on? In Western society, medical and welfare discourses would play the key role in the construction of these differences, but not entirely independently of older ideas about the body, particularly religious discourses and other cosmologies.

This is precisely the approach taken by Janet Price and her co-writers, particularly Margrit Shildrick (Potts and Price 1995; Price 1996; Shildrick and Price 1996; Price and Shildrick 1998, see also Shildrick 1997). As a feminist author who writes in her personal experience of living with a diagnosis of ME, Price, together with her co-writers, applies postmodernist perspectives to the analysis of disability, impairment and the body: 'both the disability rights movement and feminism have largely declined to come to terms with the admittedly risky strategies offered by postmodernism, preferring instead to address the issues from within familiar paradigms' (Price and Shildrick 1998: 225) (on postmodernism, see Chapter 7). The suggestion is that the body itself is constructed and maintained as disabled or non-disabled, impaired or non-impaired:

> The postmodernist claim that there is no essential biologically given corpus upon which meaning is inscribed, and no unmediated access to a body prior to discourse, remains contentious. It is not that the materiality of the body is in doubt, but that materiality is a process negotiated through the discursive exercise of what Foucault (1980) calls power/knowledge. To both the biomedical profession with its fantasy of descriptive objectivity, and to the [disability rights movement] with its investment in the notion that impairment can be separated off from disability, the claim is anathema. While both may subscribe to the view that healthcare practices are both normative and normalising, there is little recognition that those practices are also constitutive of the body. As Judith Butler puts it . . . 'there is no reference to a pure body which is not at the same time a further formation of that body' (1993: 10). What that means is that the physical impairments of the body, and the socially constructed disability are equally constructs held in place by the regulatory practices that both produce and govern *all* bodies.
>
> (Price and Shildrick 1998: 234)

Price and Shildrick draw heavily on Foucauldian analysis but note that the dominant discourses which constitute the 'normal body' are highly gendered: Foucault's referent is always the healthy *male* body. They discuss the gendered character of the disciplinary and regulatory practices in biomedicine and welfare systems which construct and control the impaired and disabled body (Shildrick and Price 1996). For Price and her co-authors, the boundaries of 'sameness' and 'difference' are not fixed but are fluid and continually in the process of construction and maintenance through discursive practices and performativity. This means that identity cannot be read off from stable or static social 'types', categories, or 'signifiers' such as 'impaired' or 'disabled'. There are no binary divides: disabled/non-disabled; impaired/non-impaired; female/male; black/white.

Another British-based writer who adopts a deconstructionist perspective is Mairian Corker (1997; 1998a; 1998b; Corker and French 1999), whose work was introduced in Chapter 3. Corker describes herself as a sociolinguist and a feminist, and the focus of her research is the relationship between Deaf people, deaf people, and the disabled people's movement.[3] Drawing on personal experiences as a deaf woman and on the work of Foucault and poststructuralists such as Derrida and Ricoeur, Corker explores the constructions and politics of the Deaf community, deafness and disability. Corker points out that Deaf people (that is, those who identify themselves as belonging to Deaf culture) do not see themselves or other deaf people as impaired or disabled. That deaf people are included among 'the impaired' flows, in the Deaf view, from phonocentrism – the dominant culture's belief in the superiority of spoken languages. Phonocentrism was firmly established in nineteenth-century Western culture and is a key discursive practice in the oppression of deaf people.

Corker argues against what she sees as the essentialism of *both* social modellists in the disabled people's movement *and* Deaf activists in Deaf communities. Both groups construct absolutes and either/or distinctions: on the one hand social modellists say that 'socio-structural barriers create disability', on the other Deaf activists assert 'we are Deaf – a minority language group – not disabled'. From a poststructuralist perspective, Corker argues that like other absolutes and binaries these cannot be sustained: meanings are never fixed but evolve and change. In championing their own concerns, both groups create new discourses, and each discourse serves to marginalize and exclude particular 'Others'. Thus she argues that the social modellist's disability discourse operates to exclude those groups for whom language and communication are critical in some way, and this is perpetuated by the disabled people's movement's disinterest in the role of culture and discourse in the construction of disability. In her work, Corker charts an interesting path between the Deaf and disabled worlds, but also bridges them. She has a strong political allegiance to the anti-discrimination campaigns of both whilst at the same time critiquing the discursive practices evident in each.

Identity

What is the relationship between identity (self-identity and ascribed identity) and the kinds of 'differences' discussed? And what are the implications for disability politics? The writings of Susan Wendell, Jenny Morris, Janet Price and her co-writers, and Mairian Corker, lead to different ways of understanding the connection between 'who we are' (the ontological status of being) and 'who we think we are' (our self-identity).

Identity politics

Jenny Morris sees her identity as being fundamentally bound up with having an impaired body (seen as an 'essential' difference), as well as being a disabled person and a woman (seen as socially constructed differences). These differences are celebrated (Morris 1991). Morris sees no difficulty in referring to other disabled women as being 'like' her and unlike non-disabled people, and she readily uses the terms 'we', 'us' and 'them'. For Morris, therefore, one's identity can be 'read off' from the categories to which one belongs: impaired, disabled, woman, white, or whatever. I will refer to this as a *categorical* approach to identity (Somers 1994). Identity politics is a relatively unproblematic option, but rather than support the notion of a fragmented set of social movements, Morris is a strong supporter of the disabled people's movement (disability identity being key). However, she asserts that unity around the issues of disability rights and disability culture should accommodate, and certainly not ignore or silence, other differences associated with gender, 'race' and so on.

Susan Wendell is more cautious but nevertheless shares features of Morris's categorical approach. Very aware of the danger of false universalisms, Wendell weighs up the pros and cons of saying that there is or can be an individual and/or collective experience which constitutes the basis for a 'disabled identity'. As noted earlier, she suggests that whilst being disabled does not, in itself, give a person a particular point of view or self-identity, there are nevertheless differences in experience which endow epistemic advantages:

> I want to say that having a disability usually gives a person experiences of the world different from people without disabilities, and that being a woman with a disability usually gives a person different experiences from those who are not disabled and female.
>
> (Wendell 1996: 73)

Wendell concludes, with qualifications, that disabled people do have a different 'standpoint', or rather standpoints, associated both with essential (impairment-related) and socially constructed differences. These, and other standpoints connected with the categories of 'race', class, sexuality, age and so on, are seen to be the fragments which make up a fractured self-identity, and which can underpin collective identities and identity politics.

Categorical approaches suffer from the paradox, referred to earlier, that by identifying with and celebrating their 'difference' disabled people might reinforce and sustain (rather than challenge) categories which have been socially produced within an oppressive disablist and patriarchal society. In addition, they can easily be used to support mechanically reductionist and ahistorical notions that there are fixed categories which produce fixed identities, for example, that 'being disabled' is an unchanging, transhistorical phenomenon which always and everywhere gives rise to the same 'disabled identity'. I am not suggesting that this is what Morris and Wendell do, but simply pointing out a danger inherent in categorical approaches.

Margaret Somers (1994: 611–12) helpfully sums up some of the difficulties with categorical approaches to identity, focusing on gender issues:

> a gender centred identity politics does not take on the real challenge of criticizing, contesting, transforming, indeed escaping from the theoretical dichotomies that buttress and hierarchize forms of difference in the first place. Instead, the new identity theories reify anew what is in fact a multiplicity of historically varying forms of what are less often unified and singular and more often 'fractured identities'. Thus although some scholars claim that establishing an identity or expressing self-realization is one of the goals of new social movements, there are others who consider the newly celebrated but fixed categories of identity and self-realization to be newly problematic, regardless of their being informed by the traits of the previously excluded.

The instability of 'identity'

Do deconstructionist perspectives like those of Price and her co-workers and Corker, offer a better way of understanding identity? They reject notions that identity is made up of categories such as 'disabled/non-disabled', 'impaired/non-impaired', 'straight/lesbian', 'black/white' and so on, because these categories, and the boundaries which demarcate them, are seen to be constituted through discursive practices, and thus are not 'real'. Identity cannot simply be 'read off' from being 'disabled', 'black', a 'woman'. And logically, there is no question of there being an 'epistemic advantage' associated with being impaired or disabled because there are no 'essential' differences which could found it. Rather, to maintain any sense of 'who I am' one has to participate constantly in the process of constructing and reconstructing the boundaries of the self through an ongoing process of differentiating oneself from 'the Other'. One cannot just 'be' something or someone because one's beingness has to be 'performed' if it is to have any existence at all, and so identity is always unstable and insecure. Identity politics is thus seen to be highly problematic.

For anti-essentialists there cannot be an identity politics; indeed, identity politics is seen as reinscribing the very boundaries it seeks to challenge:

> If our self-identity is provisional and unstable, identity politics breaks down, for it is not possible to identify a fixed unifying factor, whether material or discursive, that brings such an apparently disparate group together within, for example, the disabled people's or the women's health movement.
>
> (Price 1996: 44)

What kinds of politics or radicalism are possible? What is needed, it is suggested, is a move beyond identity politics towards a 'radical destabilization of categories', that is, the exposure of the fluid and culturally constituted character of apparently fixed categories through their deconstruction and counter-performance. At least at an individual level, 'transgressive resistance' can be displayed:

> The discontinuities continually break through, opening up a gap between bodily form, appearance, function and ability: the deaf person who can hear you perfectly, till you turn your back on them; the woman who uses a wheelchair and has just qualified as an aerobics instructor; the visually impaired woman who greets you in the evening on the street but cannot see you in the light of day. These disruptions speak not to the apparent limits of an impaired body, but rather break with the normative identities of those who are blind, deaf, disabled and so on.
>
> (Shildrick and Price 1996: 107)

Thus a new type of radicalism is believed to be possible, involving the purposive disruption of the boundaries, the problematization of identity, the destabilization of binaries and fixities: 'A more radical politics of disability, then, would disrupt the norms of dis/abled identity, not by pluralising the conditions of disability . . . but rather by exposing the failure of those norms to ever fully and finally contain a definitive standard' (Price and Shildrick 1998: 236).

It is interesting that Price is reflexively open about the tensions and personal dilemmas that she feels in rejecting the possibility of political movements based on identity categories. She states that she does not want to deny the importance of the women's health movement or the disabled people's movement, and in the final analysis appears to leave the options open (Price 1996). In their later writing, Price and Shildrick are careful to explain that they are not offering 'ultimate political solutions', and in an apparently contradictory move also state that they advocate the use of the social model of disability despite its essentialist mirroring of the medical model.

Reflecting on the debates about difference

In this chapter we have seen how the essentialism/constructionism distinction offers an approach which can be effectively applied in the process of unpacking, and differentiating between, the analyses of feminist writers in Disability Studies. Interesting and important insights and ways of seeing have been brought to light concerning the nature of difference, disability, impairment, identity and politics. However, having used this distinction, I now want to discuss what I see as the limits to the usefulness of this approach. This is where my materialism most clearly sets me apart from feminists who work within postmodernist frameworks.

Diana Fuss's distinction between essentialist and constructionist analyses of gender, sex and other differences, outlined at the start of this chapter, expresses a paradigmatic analytical opposition which now appears axiomatic in much feminist debate about difference. As indicated, this distinction has emerged in the wake of the rise of postmodernist perspectives in the social sciences and humanities. Essentialism is 'classically defined as a belief in true essence – that which is most irreducible, unchanging and therefore constitutive of a given person or thing' (Fuss 1989: 2), and is found in those explanations for gender (or other social) differences which resort to ideas about underlying 'pre-social' or biological differences. Constructionists, on the other hand, 'take the refusal of essence as the inaugural moment of their own projects and proceed to demonstrate the way previously assumed self-evident kinds (like "man" or "woman") are in fact the effects of complicated discursive practices' (Fuss 1989: 2). As Fuss points out, for many feminists essentialism is held to be 'bad', a modernist hang-over to be avoided at all costs, whilst constructionism, or relativism, is 'good'. Thus, to say that an author has an essentialist approach is often taken to mean that they are automatically in error. Fuss identifies herself as a constructionist who shares with other anti-essentialists an eagerness to avoid 'the dangers of positing natural explanations for sociopolitical effects' (Fuss 1989: 51), but her main argument is an interesting one, and indicates that the essentialist/constructionist dualism is itself problematic. It is that 'social constructionists do not definitively escape the pull of essentialism, that indeed essentialism subtends the very idea of constructionism' (Fuss 1989: 5). In fact, constructionism 'really operates as a more sophisticated form of essentialism' (Fuss 1989: xii). In making her case, she exposes the ill-founded nature of seeing essentialism and constructionism as absolutely counterposed; she asserts that, in and of itself, 'essentialism is neither good nor bad, progressive nor reactionary, beneficial nor dangerous' (Fuss 1989: xi).

In my view there are other problems with the essentialism/constructionism distinction. The main difficulty is that this new dualism serves to elide any explanatory approach which seeks to be materialist, or realist, *but not* biologically or socially reductionist. It is just such an approach that I want to pursue in the next chapter. Those who hold to an essentialism/constructionism world-view adopt the position that not to be a constructionist is inevitably to be a reductionist – there is nothing in between (see the discussion of the foundations of postmodernist thinking in the next chapter). In my view, 're-actionary' naturalistic, biologically reductionist arguments (biologism, or sociobiology) do not follow inexorably from the premise, which I support, that there are *real* biological (genetic, morphological, anatomical) differences, or variations, among people which are shaped and changed over time through the dynamic interface of the material body with the social and physical environment (and thus are not fixed and transhistorical), *some of which* have come to be culturally named and understood, through scientific medical discourses, as 'impairments' and 'abnormalities'. What is needed for the theorization of the bio-social interface, and related cultural processes, is a non-reductionist materialist ontology of the body. Thus, there are other theoretical options to constructionism which avoid the dangers of 'positing natural explanations for sociopolitical effects' (Fuss 1989: 51). Having said that, it is true, as not only postmodernists in Disability Studies have pointed out, that the social model of disability as it is currently formulated posits a naturalistic stance towards impairment, relegating it to the realm of fixed, naturally occurring, biological phenomena.

Having earlier identified their 'essentialism', it should now be clear that I have more in common with the approaches of Susan Wendell and Jenny Morris, discussed above, than with the deconstructionist perspectives of Janet Price and Margrit Shildrick, and Mairian Corker. Postmodernist approaches certainly compel us to question and unpack taken-for-granted features of culture and discourse, and this is of great value, but, in my view, the scepticism and relativism of deconstructionism are ultimately unhelpful, and its lack of explanatory power frustrating. Why, for example, do the discourses which construct the binary divisions 'disabled/non-disabled', 'impaired/non-impaired' exist? To say that these are about what Foucault calls power/knowledge is just to push the question further back: why do these power/knowledge dynamics and processes exist in society?

Of course, to ask this kind of question is, from a postmodernist perspective, to repeat the modernist error of looking for universal truth claims and falling back on macro-theoretical approaches. Constructionist approaches certainly offer important correctives to those mechanistic and reductionist materialist approaches which suggest that knowledge categories directly reflect reality without any social mediation, but, as will be discussed in the following chapter, they rest on philosophical foundations which I do not support. As Raymond Williams (1979: 167) put it: 'to recall an absolutely founding presumption of materialism . . . the material world exists whether anyone signifies it or not'.

What about identity?

In adopting an approach to impairment and disability which combines a non-reductionist materialist ontology of the body with the social relational understanding of disability outlined in Part I, what theoretical understanding of identity is required? And what kind of politics is implied? Here, I can only offer some preliminary thoughts. In contrast to both categorical and deconstructionist approaches discussed earlier, a materialist ontology would suggest that it is possible to have a consciousness of self, a subjectivity, which is on the one hand forged in the interaction between one's 'real' body and the 'real' physical and social environments in which it exists, *and* on the other hand has the capacity to act as a force upon and for itself. That is, as well as being socially produced, our subjectivities involve a psyche which can 'receive something from the outside then make it its own, thus creating something different' (Craib 1997: 5). Such a self would not be passively constructed, nor 'read off' from particular categories or attributes which appear to describe one's social status, nor a fiction or an imaginary quality in a constant state of instability.

The feminist philosopher, Morwenna Griffiths (1995), offers an interesting metaphor for identity formation: the spider's web. This captures the perspective that identity is both socially produced and self-constructed:

> Spiders make webs which are nearly invisible until the dew falls on them. They are made with threads stronger than steel and take their shape from the surrounding circumstances and from the spider herself. Second, women have traditionally made webs: knitting, tapestry, crochet and lace. Their creations are constrained by the circumstances of their making but they bear the mark of the maker. They can, like Penelope in the Odyssey, untangle the webs they have made for their own reasons and to suit their own purposes . . . [Webs are] intricate, involved, interlaced, with each part entangled with the rest and dependent on it . . . The idea of the web can throw light on the idea of the self and its politics. It, too, is made of nearly invisible, very strong threads attached to the circumstances of its making and under the control of its maker. It, too, is made to suit the purposes of its maker, but the circumstances of the making are not under her control. It, too, can be thought of as fragments in a conglomeration, or as a unitary whole; though whether it is a whole, or which whole it is, depends on the viewer as much as on its own constitution. It, too, is intricate, entangled and interlaced, with each part connected to other parts. A value of this metaphor is its flexibility. Looked at in some ways, the self is like the whole web. Looked at in others, it is like the nodes where the lines cross, or where the individual stitches resolve themselves into patterns and pictures as a result of the other individual stitches.
>
> (Griffiths 1995: 2)[4]

Elaborating this theme, Griffiths utilizes the idea that identity is *narratively* constructed. Others have followed a similar path when thinking about self-identity and its construction (Shakespeare 1996a). For example, in his deliberations on self-identity, the sociologist, Anthony Giddens, states that '[s]elf-identity . . . is not just something that is just given, as a result of the continuities of the individual's action-system, but something that has to be routinely created and sustained in the reflexive activities of the individual' (Giddens 1991: 52), and goes on to suggest that:

> [a] person's identity is not to be found in behaviour, nor – important though this is – in the reactions of others, but in the capacity to keep a particular narrative going. The individual's biography, if she is to maintain regular interaction with others in the day-to-day world, cannot be wholly fictive. It must continually integrate events which occur in the external world, and sort them into an ongoing 'story' about the self.
>
> (Giddens 1991: 54)

On the significance of narrative in identity formation, the work of Margaret Somers (1994; Somers and Gibson 1994) is particularly helpful:[5]

scholars are postulating something much more substantive about narrative: namely, that social life is itself *storied* and that narrative is an *ontological condition of social life*. Their research is showing that stories guide action; that people construct identities (however multiple and changing) by locating themselves or being located within the repertoire of emplotted stories; that 'experience' is constituted through narratives; that people make sense of what has happened and is happening to them by attempting to assemble or in some way to integrate these happenings within one or more narratives; and that people are guided to act in certain ways, and not others, on the basis of the projections, expectations, and memories derived from a multiplicity but ultimately limited repertoire of available social, public, and cultural narratives.

(Somers 1994: 613–14)

Somers uses the concept of *narrative identity* to capture this storied quality of self-identity, and locates 'ontological narratives' in the context of surrounding 'public narratives' and 'metanarratives'. She presents a strong case for a narrative identity approach in opposition both to the 'categorical' approaches to identity characteristic of academic work on identity politics and to past sociological antipathy both to 'narrative' (because of its 'discursive', 'non-explanatory' and 'non-theoretical' associations) as well as to the topics of 'being' and identity (seen as the domain of psychologists and philosophers). Her argument is that the narrative concept should be reframed so as to highlight its epistemological and ontological significance:

These [new approaches to narrative] posit that it is through narrativity that we come to know, understand, and make sense of the world, and it is through narratives and narrativity that we constitute our social identities . . . [All] of us come to be who we *are* (however ephemeral, multiple, and changing) by being located or locating ourselves (usually unconsciously) in social narratives *rarely of our own making*.

(Somers 1994: 606)

The narrative identity approach allows Somers, like Griffiths, to see identity as both socially produced in particular historical times and places, and to be acted upon and shaped by the individual: 'A narrative identity approach assumes that social action can only be intelligible if we recognise that people are guided to act by the structural and cultural relationships in which they are embedded and by the stories through which they constitute their identities' (Somers 1994: 625).

This approach allows us to identify the ways in which ontological narratives are constituted through public narratives and metanarratives, in the context of the unfixed and changing, but nevertheless 'real', structural and cultural relationships in which people are embedded. It is a conceptual approach which, because it allows for agency, enables us to see how collective identity and political change are possible. *Counter-narratives* belonging to the socially excluded and the socially marginalized emerge as critiques of the dominant public narratives, and if these counter-narratives reach excluded individuals then these individuals may change their ontological narratives and come to actively identify with others so rescripted. A new social movement becomes a possibility. So, '[s]truggles over narrations are thus struggles over identity' (Somers 1994: 631).

Endings

The disabled people's movement, with its 'social model of disability', offers a counter-narrative which has enabled many disabled people (including myself) to construct a new ontological narrative and to identify with other disabled people in a collective political struggle for disability rights and cultural change. In this view, one does not identify oneself as 'disabled' simply because one *is* 'disabled' or 'impaired' in a categorical or essentialist sense, but because one set of strands in one's web of identity – or one chapter in one's ontological narrative – has been subjectively acted upon, rewoven, and retold in the light of counter-narratives. Other counter-narratives which contest the public narratives of gender, 'race', sexuality, age and so on are also of critical importance to the many disabled people who are marginalized in other ways – because they are women, black, gay, older and so on. These make up other elements of their self-identities, but they do not exist in separate psychic departments and so cannot be seen as outside, or nothing to do with, disability politics. On the contrary, they suffuse and thus enrich disability politics: 'Oppressed people resist by identifying themselves as subjects, by defining their reality, shaping their new identity, naming their history, telling their story' (bell hooks, cited in Plummer 1995: 30).

Having examined issues of gender, disability, impairment, and 'difference' in this and the other chapters in Part II, the scene is now set for the further consideration of theoretical matters in Part III.

Notes

1 For example: on gender, see Morris (1991; 1993a; 1993b; 1995; 1996) and Begum (1992); on sexuality, see Appleby (1994), Corbett (1994), Shakespeare *et al.* (1996), Shakespeare (1997b); on 'race' and ethnicity, see Stuart (1993), Begum *et al.* (1994), Priestley (1995), Vernon (1996; 1997); on age, see Zarb and Oliver (1992), Kennedy (1996), Morris (1997), Robinson and Stalker (1998).

2 I noted in Chapter 1 that Tom Shakespeare has recently taken issue with the view that Disability Studies continues to ignore disabled women and issues of gender, arguing that, in fact, it is disabled men's experiences which are now under-represented (Shakespeare 1996b).

3 On Corker's distinctions between 'Deaf' and 'deaf', see Chapter 3, note 7.

4 This echoes Marx's famous statement, see Chapter 7 (see Marx, 1972: 10).

5 I used Somer's approach in my chapter on *Narrative Identity and the Disabled Self*, in Corker and French's *Disability Discourse* (Thomas 1999).

PART III

UNDERSTANDING DISABILITY

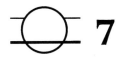 **7**

Theorizing disability and impairment

Introduction

This chapter provides an overview of theoretical work on the nature of disability and impairment within British Disability Studies. It also outlines my own thoughts on this work and the ways that disability theory can be taken forward. In so doing, it draws together the conceptual threads woven through earlier chapters, especially: the need for a social relational definition of disability, the need to theorize impairment, impairment effects and their interaction with disability, and the need to understand disability as a gendered phenomenon. The chapter begins with a summary of what has been said on these conceptual threads in preceding chapters. This is followed in the subsequent two sections by brief, and necessarily limited, outlines of two theoretical paradigms and their applications: historical materialism and postmodernism. These paradigms are particularly influential in Disability Studies at present, but, as I have already made clear in this book, my own theoretical perspective owes much more to the former than to the latter. The final section reflects on the ways forward.

Disability and impairment

Disability

In preceding chapters I have argued that a social relational definition of disability should be the starting point for the development of disability theory. In Chapter 2 the social relational understanding of disability – wherein disability is conceptualized as the social imposition of restrictions of activity on people with impairments – was distinguished from the property approach – wherein disability is thought of as restrictions of activity experienced by people with impairment which are then causally attributed to social barriers.

The social relational formulation indicates that the term disability expresses an unequal power relationship between those who are socially constructed as 'impaired' (the relatively powerless) and those who are identified as 'non-impaired' or 'normal' in society (the relatively powerful). Thus, in the same way that the concept of patriarchy refers to the relationship of male domination over women, so the concept of disability refers to the relationship of domination of the non-impaired over the impaired. But how can this relationship be understood and explained? Is it a timeless, transhistorical phenomenon, or a relationship that takes different forms in particular times and places? In Chapter 3, the social relational approach was extended so that the psycho-emotional dimensions of disability could be encompassed, and that chapter closed with a summary statement of my preferred social relational definition of disability – as a form of social oppression involving the social imposition of restrictions of activity on people with impairments and the socially engendered undermining of their psycho-emotional well-being. In Chapter 5, another and related question was posed following the observation that disability is gendered: how should the intersection, or articulation, of disability and gender oppression be theorized? To this could be added questions concerning its intersections with 'race', class, sexuality and age.

How one attempts to address the questions outlined above depends on the theoretical framework one brings to bear in making sense of the social world. I have indicated that mine is a materialist feminist perspective which means that explanations for social phenomena such as disability and women's oppression are seen to be rooted in the level of development of the productive forces, the social relations of production and reproduction, and the cultural and ideological formations in society. But what does this mean? Where does such a perspective come from? And how does it differ from other theoretical approaches? The discussion in the following two sections is designed to throw light on these matters.

Impairment

The key points made about impairment and impairment effects in previous chapters are as follows. The Introduction indicated that I do not treat 'impairment' as a self-evident given or as an unproblematized referent to 'the body' or 'the biological'. However, this does not mean that impairments are treated *only* as social constructs, as linguistic categories of meaning which bear no relationship to 'real' body-related variations. In my own usage, impairment refers to those body-related variations which in Western culture have become markers of socially, or more precisely medically, defined 'significant deviations from the normal type' or 'abnormalities'.

Chapter 1 noted that one of the themes in the emerging critique of the social model of disability is the tendency among social modellists, once they have distinguished disability from impairment, to ignore or deny the significance of impairment either for disability theory or in terms of its impact on the daily lives of disabled people. The ensuing debate, especially in relation to the personal experience of living with impairment, was discussed in some detail in Chapter 4. My argument there was that the social modellists' avoidance of matters of personal experience (whether of impairment or disability) was bound up with deeply rooted conceptual dualisms separating the personal and the political, the private and the public. I outlined my view that the personal experience of living with both disability and impairment (and the interaction of these) should be on the Disability Studies agenda.

In making the distinction between a social relational and a property conceptualization of disability in Chapter 2, I attempted to unhook disability from its equation with 'restrictions of activity' and this, in turn, made room for the idea that as well as disabilities there are also impairment effects. The introduction of this term was an acknowledgement that, from a 'disability as social relation' point of view, some restrictions of activity (that is, not being able to function in certain ways, or 'to do' certain things) *are* directly caused by physical, sensory or intellectual impairments and would not be eliminated by the cessation of disablism. It was argued that the lived experiences of disabled people are shaped in fundamental ways by the interaction of disability and impairment effects, and that Disability Studies should not eschew but take up the study of both the social dimensions of impairment and impairment effects. Chapter 2 also made the point that disability, impairment and impairment effects cannot be simply mapped on to the familiar social/biological or cultural/natural dualisms – with disability being about the social, and impairment/impairment effects being about the biological or the natural. This theme was central to the discussion in Chapter 6 where disability and impairment were considered from the perspective of feminist debates on the nature of 'difference'; discussion focused on 'essentialist' versus 'constructionist' ideas about being impaired, as represented in the work of a number of disabled feminist writers. In contrast to either essentialist or constructionist formulations, my own conclusion was that the development of a materialist ontology of impairment and impairment effects is necessary – an ontology which is neither biologically reductionist nor culturally determinist.

How can these ideas on disability and impairment be taken forward? Two theoretical perspectives of importance in contemporary Disability Studies and their applications will now be examined.

Historical materialism

The social model of disability is frequently referred to, sometimes disparagingly, as materialist. So unfashionable is Marxism in contemporary sociology and feminism generally, that knowledge about historical materialism cannot be assumed. Materialism is often wrongly equated with crude economic determinism, or economic reductionism, and with the view that individuals in society are pawns without agency. In addition, such an interpretation supposes that materialists see culture as of little or no significance, believing that everything in society is directly or mechanically determined by aspects of production. This is a misrepresentation. Of course, the work of some people who call themselves 'Marxist' has displayed this meagre version of material-ism, but it is not one which I wish to endorse here.

Interestingly, in academic texts one often comes across the following phrase, used to express the importance of examining *both* structure and agency in sociological work: 'people make their own history but not under conditions of their own choosing'. It is often forgotten, or not appreciated, that this is a paraphrase of Marx's statement in *The Eighteenth Brumaire of Louis Bonaparte*. Here it is in full (with its gendered language of the day): 'Men [*sic*] make their own history, but they do not make it just as they please; they do not make it under circumstances chosen by themselves, but under circum-stances directly encountered, given and transmitted from the past' (Marx 1972: 10). Thus, from a materialist perspective, in their lives individuals are both determined and determining.

Materialist premises

How can the historical materialist approach be outlined briefly, given that it has been the subject of hundreds of books and papers in the past? Perhaps the best way is to go back to its premises as set down by Marx and Engels themselves in their early work, *The German Ideology* (written in 1845–60).

> we must begin by stating the first premise of all human existence and, therefore, of all history . . . namely, that men must be in a position to live in order to 'make history'. But life involves before everything else eating and drinking, a habitation, clothing and many other things. The first his-torical act is thus the production of the means to satisfy these needs, the production of material life itself [i.e. the expenditure of human labour-power]. And indeed this is an historical act, a fundamental condition of all history, which today, as thousands of years ago, must daily and hourly be fulfilled merely in order to sustain human life . . . The second point is that the satisfaction of the first need (the action of satisfying, and the instrument of satisfaction which has been acquired) leads to new needs; and this production of new needs is the first historical act. . . . The third circumstance which, from the very outset, enters into historical develop-ment, is that men, who daily remake their own life, begin to make other men, to propagate their kind: the relation between man and woman, parents and children, the *family*. The family, which to begin with is the only social relationship, becomes later, when increased needs create new relations and the increased population new needs, a subordinate one . . . and must then be treated and analysed according to the existing empiri-cal data . . . These three aspects of social activity are not of course to be taken as three different stages, but as three aspects or . . . three 'moments', which have existed simultaneously since the dawn of history and the first men, and which still assert themselves in history today.
>
> (Marx and Engels 1970: 48–50)

So, the basic materialist premise is that human life, today as in the past, is fundamentally concerned with the production and enhancement of the material conditions of life, together with the production of new life – reproduction. This, in turn, requires co-operation between individuals and sustains social relationships (Marx and Engels 1970: 50). From simple co-operation there develops an ever more complex division of labour, and the emergence of property since the division of labour soon involves the unequal distribution of labour and its products (Marx and Engels 1970: 52). Particular modes of co-operation, or different forms of property relation in time and place, constitute particular modes of production: primitive communism, antiquity, slavery, feudalism, capitalism. Thus: 'In the social production of their existence, men inevitably enter into definite relations, which are independent of their will, namely relations of production appropriate to a given stage in the development of their material forces of production' (Marx 1977: 20).

For Marx and Engels, the relations of material production in any society give rise to other 'forms of intercourse' – civil society in its various stages. This involves the form of the state as well as 'different theoretical products and forms of consciousness, religion, philosophy, ethics, etc. etc.' (Marx and Engels 1970: 58). In other words, political and cultural formations are bound up with (but not directly or mechanically determined by) the processes and relations of material production. In turn, the activities undertaken in civil society can, and do, impact upon the latter.

Consciousness, ideology and cultural expressions are therefore seen as social products arising out of the social relations and real material circumstances in any mode of production. A key aspect of society's division of labour is that which separates 'mental' and 'manual' labour, enabling some people to engage exclusively in 'mental' labour: priests, scholars and so on. Once mental labour becomes the special prerogative of the minority then consciousness *appears* to be entirely independent of its material basis:

> consciousness can really flatter itself that it is really something other than consciousness of existing practice, that it really represents something without representing something real; from now on consciousness is in a position to emancipate itself from the world and to proceed to the formation of 'pure' theory, theology, philosophy, ethics, etc.
>
> (Marx and Engels 1970: 52)

This apparent independence of ideas and knowledge systems was an important contemporary issue for Marx and Engels because in *The German Ideology* they were engaged in an extended argument with *idealist* philosophers, especially German philosophers. These philosophers completely neglected the real material basis of consciousness, and rewrote history in a teleological fashion so that it was determined either by 'The Idea' (God) which worked like a hidden hand, or by other sets of autonomous political or religious ideas. In idealism, material reality becomes the product of the idea. I emphasize this point because, as we will see in the section on postmodernism below, there are very strong echoes of this earlier idealism in present-day postmodernist and poststructuralist perspectives which argue that culture produces society, or that society is nothing other than ideas held about it. Finally, for Marx and Engels (1970: 64), '[t]he ideas of the ruling class are in every epoch the ruling ideas, i.e. the class which is the ruling material force of society, is at the same time its ruling intellectual force'.

So, what does all of this mean for understanding disability in our society? If disability is a social relational phenomenon then it must, from a materialist perspective, be somehow tied in with (and explained by) contemporary social relations of production – the capitalist mode of production. Manifestations of disability – the imposition of restrictions of activity on people with impairments and the prevalence of negative ideas about impaired people which are expressed in cultural practices – must be rooted in our epoch's social relations of production and reproduction, and sustained within the present form of civil society (the state, culture, systems of knowledge). Elements of this way of approaching the theorization of disability are expressed in a helpful paper by the Australian-based writer, Brendan Gleeson (1997a). He critically reviews Disability Studies internationally, outlining and advocating the application of materialism to the study of disability as follows:

> The crucial point is that the social construction of . . . impaired people as disabled people arises, in the first instance, from the specific ways in which society organises its basic material activities (work, transport, leisure, domestic activities). Attitudes, discourses and symbolic representation are, of course, critical to the reproduction of disablement, but are themselves the product of the social practices which society undertakes in order to meet its basic material needs.
>
> (Gleeson 1997a: 194)

Consistent with the premises of Marx and Engels outlined above, Gleeson thus looks for the material basis of disability in the social relations of production. Cultural phenomena – attitudes, discourses, symbolic representation – are seen as products of more basic social practices (see also Barnes 1996; 1997a; Oliver 1996c; Priestley 1998 – discussed in Chapter 3).

Capitalism and disability

The discussion now turns to how Disability Studies writers who adopt a materialist perspective have undertaken the application of materialist premises in the study of disability and impairment. Do we find crude or sophisticated theoretical applications of materialism? I shall take the work of Mike Oliver, Brendan Gleeson and Paul Abberley as examples.

In his book *The Politics of Disablement* (1990), Oliver sets out on the road of developing a social theory of disability, but it is important to note that whilst he uses Marxist analyses of capitalist production for this purpose, he says that his approach does 'not imply the endorsement of the theory of historical materialism, nor its applicability to a proper understanding of the nature of disability' (Oliver 1990: 25). Rather, Oliver finds it necessary to combine insights from Marxism with other theoretical perspectives, particularly to understand what he calls the 'mode of thought' in any society: 'Hence the nature of disability can only be understood by using a model which takes account of both changes in the mode of production and mode of thought, and the relationship between them' (Oliver 1990: 32). In relation to the 'modes of thought' he gives particular attention to the emergence of individualism, to the pathologizing of impairments by medicine, and to the 'personal tragedy' view of disability, drawing on work which utilizes a variety of theoretical perspectives. Nevertheless, he summarizes his view on disability as follows: 'The argument suggests that the dominant view of disability as an individual, basic, medical problem is created by the productive forces, material conditions and social relations of capitalism' (Oliver 1990: 132). In his later writings, a more explicit materialist stance is evident, as in the following passage:

> Hence the economy, through both the operation of the labour market and the social organisation of work, plays a key role in producing the category disability and in determining societal responses to disabled people. Further, the oppression that disabled people face is rooted in the economic and social structures of capitalism which themselves produce racism, sexism, homophobia, ageism and disablism.
>
> (Oliver 1996c: 33)

Building on work by Finkelstein (1980), Oliver sees the changes in production which are central to the creation of contemporary disability as follows. In pre-industrial Britain production relations in agriculture and small-scale manufacture enabled people with impairments to contribute to economic production in important ways, 'In this era disabled people were regarded as individually unfortunate and not segregated from the rest of society' (Oliver 1990: 27). Oliver notes that, whilst there is a danger of idealizing the pre-industrial position of people with impairment, there is no doubt that things got decidedly worse for them when their participation in production, and as a consequence in family and community life, was undermined with the arrival of industrial production, especially large-scale factory production. Factory production separated the workplace from the home, demanded the wholesale uprooting of people and their relocation in overcrowded and insanitary urban centres, enforced attendance for long hours at the workplace, and set minimum standards for levels of dexterity and speed of work. Many people with impairments were excluded from these new forms of production and appeared to lose their usefulness: 'As a result of this, disabled people came to be regarded as a social and educational problem and more and more were segregated in institutions of all kinds including workhouses, asylums, colonies and special schools, and out of mainstream social life' (Oliver 1990: 28). Through the nineteenth and twentieth centuries the accompanying 'mode of thought' has meant that disabled people are seen as individual victims of personal tragedy whose fate is, therefore rightly, determined by medicine and the state. For Oliver, policies of deinstitutionalization in the second half of the twentieth century have not signalled an end to seg-regation – disabled people remain relatively isolated but now in 'the com-munity' setting, excluded from the mainstream of social life through the operation of numerous 'social barriers'. Brief and rather simplistic though Oliver's sketch of the impact of the development of the capitalist production upon people with impairment is (no more than a few pages in *The Politics of Disablement*), it does suggest that the social oppression of those identified as impaired by those identified as non-impaired in capitalist society might have at its sustaining foundation their disadvantaged position in, and exclusion from, material production. This has considerable explanatory potential.

It is interesting, and telling, that the history of the term 'disability' in Britain is bound up with production. Prior to the second half of the twentieth century, there was no general conception of disability as connected with a generalized range of impairments. The Poor Law (from the sixteenth to nine-teenth centuries) defined people as disabled only when they could not operate in the labour market. The link with impairment developed in the nineteenth century. Questions began to be included in the 1851 to 1911 Cen-suses, notably on blindness, and the notion that there were groups of people with different impairments but a common social character began to take hold. However, the later use of the term 'disability' in the generic sense familiar today retained its connection with men and employment – first in relation to workmen's compensation, then the War Pensions scheme in 1916, and sub-sequently in the Industrial Injuries Scheme. The term 'disabled ex-service-men' became common after the First World War, and the meaning of disability was then extended (the Royal Warrant) by using a comparison with a 'normal' person of the same age and sex in terms of the loss of faculty or limb. The Second World War saw the Tomlinson Report which led to the setting up of services associated with the 1944 Disabled Persons Employment Act – especially rehabilitation, sheltered workshops and Remploy – during a time of labour shortage. The National Assistance Act of 1948 codified this generic usage of the term disabled. Under the Act 'the disabled' were categor-ized into the sensory impaired – the blind, the partially sighted, the deaf, the hard of hearing – and the 'general classes of the physically handicapped'. What is also notable about this history of the word 'disability' is that it is a highly gendered one. The social policy focus has been on men, employment and the effects of war on servicemen. The category 'disabled woman' only seems to have appeared, in social policy terms, with the 1948 Act.[1]

The transition from feudalism to capitalism

Continuing with materialist approaches to disability, Brendan Gleeson (1993; 1997a) has offered a more developed analysis of the kind advanced by Oliver, focusing on the emergence of disability in the transition from feudalism to capitalism in England and elsewhere. In a detailed empirical examination of the processes at work, and utilizing Marxist political economy, Gleeson tracks the spread of generalized commodity production and the corresponding transformation of labour-power into a commodity. He proposes that it was in this historical context, and in the geographical spaces involved, that disability as a form of social oppression developed – bound up with the undermining of the labour-power of people with impairments in the face of the spread of wage-labour relations. Summarizing his own research, he says:

> whilst impairment was probably a prosaic feature of feudal England, disablement was not. Gleeson . . . attributes the non-disabling character of feudal English society both to a confined realm of physical interaction and, more importantly, to the relatively weak presence of commodity production. He argues that the growth of commodity relations in late feudal England (i.e. from around the 15th century) slowly eroded the labour-power of impaired people. Market relations, and the commodification of labour, introduced a social evaluation of work – the law of value – into peasant households which had heretofore been relatively autonomous production units. The increasing authority of the law of value meant the submission of peasant households to an external force (market relations) which appraised the worth of individual labour in terms of average productivity standards. From the first, this competitive, social evaluation of individual labour-power meant that 'slower', 'weaker' or more inflexible workers were devalued in terms of their potential for paid work.
>
> (Gleeson 1997a: 194–5)

Thus Gleeson's analysis suggests that disability, as a form of social oppression, belongs to particular times and places and is not a ubiquitous, transhistorical, phenomenon. He points to the economic and related social changes bound up with capitalist development which served to distinguish and separate out 'the impaired' from the 'non-impaired', which rendered the former materially dependent on the latter, and which thus constituted the material basis of the social power of the non-impaired over the impaired. Urbanization and the spatial relocation of work (in factories, workshops and so on) 'created a powerfully disabling friction in everyday life for physically impaired people' (Gleeson 1997a: 195). In my view, Gleeson's approach holds considerable promise and could be further developed in Disability Studies to good effect.

Of course it might be argued that whilst this may well explain disability in the nineteenth century, this materialist approach does not seem so relevant today when large numbers of people with impairment can, and do, sell their labour-power and engage in either material or non-material production. Perhaps their present experiences of oppression owe more to cultural or other factors than to matters of production? In my view, this way of posing the question sets up false counter-positions: first, cultural and other factors should be seen as important aspects of oppression both in the capitalist past and in the present; second, the entry of impaired people into the labour force (and into higher education and training) does not signal the abolition of the material basis of their oppression but, rather, its changing character. The latter is bound up with the development of the productive forces within capitalist societies – particularly in the last 150 years in Britain but especially in recent decades: the ongoing mechanization of labour processes; the development of computer/information technology; the ever more specialized division of labour with the expansion of non-manual work. The challenge is to apply a materialist perspective in today's conditions – something which those researching contemporary 'social barriers' in employment, education and so on, are contributing to. The reality is that people with impairments are among the most disadvantaged of paid workers, or remain shut out of the labour market – either completely excluded from the labour force or as part of the large and heterogeneous 'reserve army of labour' characteristic of an advanced capitalist economy.

Materialism and impairment

The focus now shifts to a materialist perspective on impairment. The work of Paul Abberley (1987; 1996; 1997) is most relevant here. In 1987 he argued that a theory of disability as oppression had to recognize that impairment (like disability) is social in origin. Unlike most social modellists who purposively, or by default, left impairment in the realm of 'naturally occurring biological phenomena', Abberley proposed that these biological differences are not 'natural' but socially created.

Abberley offered an account of the origin of impairment which privileges socio-economic determinants of disease and trauma as well as highlighting the interaction of the social and the biological. He pointed, for example, to the fact that hazardous environments in workplaces and communities, together with a wide range of other social risk factors, play a key health-determining role.[2] Similarly, the *social* advances in medical science create ever higher levels of impairment in the population as the life expectancy of children and adults with impairments is extended. The consumption of products also causes impairments through accidents and injuries – for example: the side-effects of prescribed drugs, the widespread use of cars and other vehicles, the use of potentially hazardous power sources and consumer durables in the home. On a global scale, many individuals are impaired as a direct result of economic and political factors which precipitate famine, malnutrition and war. However, Abberley (1987: 12) makes it clear that 'such a view does not deny the significance of germs, genes and trauma, but rather points out that their effects are only ever apparent in a real social and historical context, whose nature is determined by a complex interaction of material and non-material factors'.

In challenging a naturalistic conceptualization of impairment, Abberley forces us to think about impairment itself as a largely socially determined phenomenon, and to recognize that the forms that impairment takes are to a great extent shaped by economic and political factors and processes. Like disability, impairment has a material foundation in the relations of production and the level of development of the productive forces. In this view impairment, like disability, does not have a transhistorical or universalistic character but is historically and spatially specific: what *is* and what *counts as* impairment is always socially located, situated in time and place. In Abberley's view, this social theorizing of impairment should be linked in with the materialist theorizing of disability: 'a theory of oppression will attempt to flesh out the claim that historically specific categories of "disabled people" were constituted as a product of the development of capitalism, and its concerns with the compulsion to work' (Abberley 1987: 17).

Abberley pursues this theme in later work, restating that the conceptual natural/social dualism is erroneous and that disability theory requires a more developed analysis of the relationship between disability and impairment: 'impairment is the material substratum upon which the oppressive social structures of disablement are erected' (Abberley 1996: 63). His perspective enables him to make the important point that 'not all restrictions on human activity are oppression' (Abberley 1996: 61), that is, not all restrictions of activity are disability. This parallels my argument in Chapter 2 that a distinction needs to be made between disability and impairment effects. Abberley uses this insight to consider the position of people with impairments in hypothetical utopian societies of the future, arguing that the overcoming of disability would leave impairment effects in place: 'for impaired people the overcoming of disablement, whilst immensely liberative, would still leave an uneradicated residue of disadvantage in relation to power over the material world' (Abberley 1996: 74). This, in turn, leads Abberley into arguments against what he sees as the 'work-based' utopian vision in Marxism as well as in much feminist thinking. Nevertheless, he reiterates the need for a thoroughgoing materialist analysis of disability:

> This is by no means to deny that the origins of our oppression, even for those with jobs, lie in our historical exclusion, as a group, from access to work, nor is it to oppose campaigns for increasing access to employment. It does, however, point out that a thoroughgoing materialist analysis of disablement today must recognize that full integration of impaired people in social production can never constitute the future to which we as a movement aspire.
>
> (Abberley 1996: 76–7)

In my view, Abberley's work on impairment is important. His analysis has exposed the biological reductionism in social modellist treatments of impairment, and pointed out that impairment is, in large measure, a social phenomenon because it is socially produced, involving the interaction of real biological and social factors (see also Wendell 1996). However, to emphasize the social creation of impairment does not fully meet the challenge of theorizing the bio-social interface – something which a materialist perspective needs to do. How are bodily variations, which in our culture come to be understood through medical discourses as 'impairments' (pathologized morphological, anatomical, genetic 'differences'), shaped and changed in time and place through the *dynamic* interrelationship between human bodies and the social and physical environments? This question has not been explored by anyone in any detail.

Perhaps a starting point would be to completely rethink the interactive relationship between human genotypes and phenotypes and the 'natural' and social environment, in historical time and space?[3] In any event, innovative, materialistically informed theoretical work is required, and at the very least it is important to avoid seeing the 'biological' simply as a fixed and unchanging bedrock upon which social processes are played out.

Materialism, gender and disability

The theorization of the intersection of disability and gender from a materialist perspective is largely uncharted territory. Some may explain this as a purportedly inevitable result of materialism's masculinist failure to address gender divisions (or any social divisions other than class), whilst for others it is simply a matter of work left undone. I take the latter view, thus not subscribing to the position that historical materialism is inherently unable to analyse gender relations, or incapable of examining the intersection of gender and disability. Rather, insights from feminist theory need to be brought together with materialist premises. On the other hand, and as discussed in Chapter 4, it is unfortunately the case that non-disabled feminists of materialist (and other theoretical) persuasions have ignored disability and the lives of disabled women.

In Chapter 5 the problems of a simplistic 'double oppression' perspective (that is, Sexism + Disablism = Double oppression) were noted, and the question was posed: if disability is rooted in the level of development of the productive forces, the social relations of production and reproduction, and the socio-cultural and ideological formations in society, then how does disability articulate with gender relations which are similarly rooted? And how should intersections with other dimensions of social division and difference be dealt with: sexuality, class, age and so forth? The best attempt to begin to theorize this from a materialist, or more accurately a socialist feminist, standpoint is found in the US-based work of Michelle Fine and Adrienne Asch (1988), briefly discussed in Chapter 5. Their edited collection considers the material and cultural locations of disabled women in contemporary industrial society, drawing attention to the fact that disabled women are more disadvantaged than either non-disabled women or disabled men. Attention is paid to the marginalized social positioning of disabled women in paid and unpaid work, in family, friendship and sexual relations, in education, in welfare, in reproduction, in political movements, in literature, and in other cultural domains. Jenny Morris's work (especially 1991; 1993a; 1993b; 1995; 1996) is also relevant, though I doubt that she would associate her approach with materialism. However, path-breakers such as Fine and Asch (1988) and Morris have been faced first and foremost with getting disabled women on to the map, and with beginning the task of documenting their experiences of disadvantage in all areas of social life. Whilst disabled women clearly emerge from this kind of research as a particularly and specifically oppressed social group, the theorization of this oppression remains in its early stages.

What are the theoretical challenges from a materialist feminist point of view? One task is to subject the analysis of the materialist roots of disability (discussed above) to a feminist critique. We know from much feminist scholarship that the histories of men and women both before and after the rapid spread of wage-labour relations during early industrial capitalism, and in the course of nineteenth-century capitalist development, are not the same. We know that women's lives in general were, and continue to be, profoundly bound up with reproduction, the performance of household labour, and. childrearing. The domestic realm was an expanding sphere of social production (unpaid labour) in the second half of the nineteenth century such that by the turn of the century only one in ten married women were in paid employment (Thomas 1996). In the twentieth century, particularly the second half, there have been very significant changes in the social position of women, associated in particular with the large-scale entry of women into paid work and into further education (see, for example, Walby 1990; 1997). So, how have disabled women fared in these gender transformations, and what have been the key gender differences? Little is known. Even less is understood about the material basis of disabled women's oppression than about disabled men's. A huge research agenda begins to open up. At the very least, there is a need to theorize the social position of women with impairments in connection with *both* production and reproduction. As Engels (1972: 71–2; emphasis added) put it in this well-known passage:

> According to the materialist conception, the determining factor in history is, in the final instance, the production *and reproduction* of immediate life. This, again, is of a twofold character: on the one side, the production of the means of existence, of food, or clothing and shelter and the tools necessary for that production; on the other side, the production of human beings themselves, the propagation of the species. The social organisation under which people of a particular country live is determined by both kinds of production: by the stage of development of labour on the one hand and by the family on the other.

However, as well as theorizing the social position of disabled women in relation to the social relations of production and reproduction, and both disablism and patriarchy, attention has to be paid to the cultural and ideological dimensions of their oppression. It is to matters of culture that I now turn.

The death of the grand narratives: postmodernism

Postmodernism and poststructuralism

For a great many social analysts today historical materialist perspectives have, along with the Marxist political programme, been relegated to the dustbins of history. Lyotard (1984) talks of the death of the metanarratives in postmodern society. Postmodernists and poststructuralists see the 'grand narratives' of the modernist epoch in Western culture, including historical materialism, as no longer of relevance except as systems of knowledge to deconstruct.[4] The search for 'universal truth claims' and for unequivocal meanings is abandoned as an Enlightenment illusion, and for many a philosophical idealist perspective is positively embraced. The French philosophers of the 1960s – especially Deleuze, Derrida, Foucault and Lyotard – have been particularly influential, schooled in the structuralism of Ferdinand de Saussure and Claude Lévi-Strauss (Lechte 1994; Cahoone 1996). Lawrence Cahoone, whose helpful introduction to his anthology, *From Modernism to Postmodernism* (1996), I draw upon quite heavily, traces the influences as follows:

> Structuralism rejected the focus on the self and its historical development that had characterised Marxism, existentialism, phenomenology, and psychoanalysis. The social or human sciences, like anthropology, linguistics, and philosophy, needed to focus instead on the super-individual structures of language, ritual, and kinship which make the individual what he or she is. Simply put, it is not the self that creates culture, but culture that creates the self. The study of abstract relations within systems or 'codes' of cultural signs . . . [viz. signs like 'disability' or 'impairment'] is the key to understanding human existence . . . [These new theorists] applied the structural-cultural analysis of human phenomena to the human sciences themselves, which are, after all, human cultural constructions. Hence they are best named 'poststructuralists'. The import of their work appeared radical indeed. They seemed to announce the end of rational inquiry into truth, the illusory nature of any unified self, the impossibility of clear and unequivocal meaning, the illegitimacy of western civilisation, and the oppressive nature of all modern institutions.
>
> (Cahoone 1996: 5–6)

In bringing about this shift, such that cultural matters or 'cultural discourses' are seen as determining of self and society, the writings of the linguist, Saussure, have been particularly influential. In Saussure's theory of language there is no essential bond between word (signifier) and thing (signified), and language is thus relatively autonomous of reality; further, the relationship between the signifier and the signified is arbitrary:

> With the emergence of the Sassurian model in the human sciences, the researcher's attention was turned away from documenting historical events, or recording the facts of human behaviour, and towards the notion of human action as a system of meaning. . . . Whereas the search for intrinsic facts and their effects had hitherto been made (as exemplified when the historian supposed that human beings need food to survive, just as they need language to communicate with each other – therefore events turned out this way), now the socio-cultural system at a given moment in history, becomes the object of study.
>
> (Lechte 1994: 151)

These kinds of ideas have had a major impact in feminism and sociology (the emergence of deconstructionism, the cultural or linguistic 'turn' in the social sciences generally), and, as evidenced in Chapters 1, 3 and 6, are increasingly drawn upon in Disability Studies (see especially Price 1996; Shakespeare 1996a; 1997a; Shildrick and Price 1996; Hughes and Paterson 1997; Corker 1998a; 1998b; Price and Shildrick 1998; Corker and French 1999). Disability and impairment become matters of culture – cultural signs, linguistic signifiers, discourses which constitute people's reality. There is no 'underlying material reality'.

Another key influence is the work of Michel Foucault (1967; 1972; 1973; 1977; 1979–86) which has been widely embraced, especially his theory of the domination of bodies through techniques tied up with the operation of 'truth games' or powerful cultural discourses (for example, professional discourses in biology, psychiatry, medicine) which are imposed by others and then become self-imposed. In this view, disabled people are oppressively disciplined by medical and welfare discourses in contemporary culture, and come to discipline themselves since their worlds are constituted through discursive practices (see especially Shildrick and Price 1996, discussed in Chapter 6). However, in his (sympathetic) discussion about Foucault's and others' theories of 'the body', Arthur Frank (1991: 57) makes an important point about the apparent absence of agency in Foucault's analysis:

> The problem with such a truth game as a model of social power is that she who is subject to the truth game is, to rephrase Garfinkel's famous charge against Parsons, a 'discourse dope'. What is difficult to theorize is how players can be dominated but not be dopes.

Are disabled people passive victims of disciplinary control? This seems to be the implication in some Foucauldian Disability Studies analyses.

Moving on, any suggestion that disability is rooted in the level of development of the productive forces, the social relations of production and reproduction is anathema to postmodernist thought, not only because the statement does not restrict itself to matters of cultural meaning but because to suggest that we can get to the root or 'origin' of something is, supposedly, a modernist fallacy. As Cahoone (1996: 15) puts it:

> Postmodernism denies the possibility of returning to, recapturing, or even representing the origin, source, or any deeper reality behind phenomena, and casts doubt on or even denies its existence. In a sense, postmodernism is intentionally superficial, not through eschewing rigorous analysis, but by regarding the surface of things, the phenomena, as not requiring a reference to anything deeper or more fundamental. . . . postmodernism tries to show that what others have regarded as a unity, a single, integral existence or concept, is plural. This is to some extent a reflection of structuralism, which understood cultural elements – words, meanings, experiences, human selves, societies – as constituted by relations to other elements. Since such relations are inevitably plural, the individual in question is plural as well. Everything is constituted by

relations to other things, hence nothing is simple, immediate, or totally present, and no analysis of anything can be complete or final.

Thus what is required, in the study of disability or anything else, is a purposive conceptual privileging of surface appearance, a flexibility and openness to plurality.

Another characteristic feature of postmodernist thought which, in Disability Studies, has been utilized particularly by Tom Shakespeare (1997a; see Chapter 3), and Janet Price and Margrit Shildrick (Price 1996; Shildrick and Price 1996; Price and Shildrick 1998; see Chapters 3 and 6): is the idea of 'constitutive otherness' in analysing cultural entities. Cahoone (1996: 16) explains this concept as follows:

> What appear to be cultural units – human beings, words, meanings, ideas, philosophical systems, social organizations [viz. 'normal' people] – are maintained in their apparent unity only through an active process of exclusion, opposition, and hierarchization. Other phenomena or units [viz. impaired people] must be represented as foreign or 'other' through representing a hierarchical dualism in which the unit is 'privileged' or favored, and the other is devalued in some way. For example, in examining social systems characterized by class or ethnic division, postmodernists will discover that the privileged groups must actively produce and maintain their position by representing or picturing themselves – in thought, in literature, in law, in art – as not having the properties ascribed to the under-privileged groups, and must represent those groups as lacking the properties of the privileged groups. . . . Only in this way can the pristine integrity of the idealized or privileged term be maintained.

In my view, this constitutive otherness idea is both interesting and useful, and certainly draws attention to the cultural forces continually at work in representing disabled people (black people, 'gays', and so on) as 'Other' and thus as inferior.

The postmodernist challenge in Disability Studies

To some authors in Disability Studies, postmodernist and poststructuralist perspectives offer a welcome relief from what are perceived to be the narrow constraints of a dominant materialist social model. From a postmodern perspective the key weaknesses in the latter are the social modellist tendency:

(i)   to ignore or downplay the role of culture in the oppression of disabled people with a concomitant privileging of socio-structural barriers in their analyses (Shakespeare 1996a; 1997a; Corker 1998a; Corker and French 1999);

(ii) to ignore impairment and to 'naturalize' it, that is, to see it in an 'essentialist' and biologically reductionist way (Shildrick and Price 1996; Hughes and Paterson 1997; Price and Shildrick 1998; Corker and French 1999); and

(iii) to make a rigid distinction between the personal and the political, or the realms of the private and the public, and to argue that personal and private experiences of disability and impairment are of no real concern or interest in Disability Studies and disability politics (see Shakespeare 1996a; 1997a; Corker and French 1999). Each of these points will be discussed in turn.

Culture

The criticism that materialistically inclined social modellists have ignored or downplayed cultural processes was discussed in Chapter 3, and certainly has some weight. I will not repeat that discussion here, but draw attention to the fact that more is at issue in the debate than simply the importance of giving due weight and consideration to culture. In other words, postmodernists are saying much more than that materialists should place culture more prominently in their analyses (something I can readily agree with). What is being claimed is that culture is pre-eminent, there *is only* culture (at least for a consistent postmodernist). From the outline of postmodernist and poststructuralist perspectives above, it is clear that cultural processes are overwhelmingly privileged. For poststucturalists, social life is understood entirely in terms of meanings, discourses, discursive practices, and the constitution of experience through language. If culture is seen to create the self, then 'disabled people' and 'impaired people' are not 'givens', but are neither more nor less than linguistically and discursively created categories whose categorical boundaries have to be continually reproduced through discursive practices, including 'constitutive othering'. It is inherent in the logic of postmodernism that the traditional social modellist preoccupation with the social imposition of structural barriers in employment, education, the built environment, and so on, is of little or no intellectual interest. Nor is there any point in searching for 'the roots' or 'causes' of disability in relations of production or anywhere else because such an enterprise belongs to a bygone Enlightenment fixation with linear causal processes and the search for universal truth claims. It is this overwhelming emphasis on culture, together with the freeing of cultural processes from any kind of material foundation, which I find most problematic about postmodernist approaches. Nonetheless, those using postmodernist perspectives have assisted greatly in drawing attention to the existence and importance of powerful discourses which do play a key role in shaping disabled people's experiences: discourses in medicine, state welfare agencies, education and elsewhere.

Impairment, boundaries and dualism

In drawing attention to the culturally constituted nature of meaning and categories, postmodernist and poststructuralist approaches continually remind us not to take concepts like disability and impairment for granted, as fixed 'givens'. An argument which is increasingly heard from postmodernists (or those influenced by postmodernism) in Disability Studies is that whilst traditional social modellists have 'reauthored' the concept of disability – wrenching it from medical discourses and giving it a new meaning – they have not done the same with 'impairment':

> there is a powerful convergence between biomedicine and the social model of disability with respect to the body. Both treat it as a pre-social, inert, physical object, as discrete, palpable and separate from the self. The definitional separation of impairment and disability which is now a semantic convention for the social model follows the traditional, Cartesian, western meta-narrative of human constitution.
>
> (Hughes and Paterson 1997: 329)

Thus it is suggested that social modellists set up an untenable dualism wherein disability belongs to the 'social' whilst impairment belongs, in an essentialist fashion, to the 'biological'; impairment is then ignored and left languishing in the modernist medical discourse, accepted as an 'abnormal' or 'deviant' biological state: 'The shift to a social oppression model of disability consigns the bodily aspects of disability to a reactionary and oppressive discursive space' (Hughes and Paterson 1997: 328).

These disability/impairment, social/biological dualisms in social modellist accounts are certainly a weakness, as already discussed, but does post-modernism provide an adequate corrective? Bill Hughes and Kevin Paterson (1997), for whom materialism is out of the question, have considered the matter in some depth and assert that Disability Studies requires a sociology of impairment which draws on Foucauldian and other poststructuralist perspectives, together with phenomenological perspectives (phenomenology is touched on in the following chapter). They turn to phenomenology for telling reasons: they are forced to acknowledge that a poststructuralist perspective on impairment is problematic because it denies the 'realness', the materiality, of the impaired body. They put it as follows:

> Post-structuralism replaces biological essentialism with discursive essentialism. The body becomes nothing more than the multiple significations that give it meaning. Post-modern consciousness actually annihilates the body as a palpable, natural material object. The body and the sensate – in effect – disappear into language and discourse, and lose their organic constitution in the pervasive sovereignty of the symbol. Foucault's concept of bio-politics robs the body of agency and renders it biologically barren. The body becomes a surface to be written on, to be fabricated by the regimes of truth . . .
>
> (Hughes and Paterson 1997: 333–4)

Whether phenomenology, with its emphasis on lived experience, holds the answer to these difficulties remains to be seen.

One of the notable features of Hughes and Paterson's (1997) analysis is that they ignore Paul Abberley's work on impairment, discussed earlier. One can only presume that Hughes and Paterson see any materialist approach to impairment as hopelessly caught up in 'western meta-narratives', and therefore not worthy of comment. But it was more than ten years ago that Abberley, a materialist, pointed to exactly the same key problem: that impairment is naturalized and ignored by social modellists. If Abberley's contribution had been discussed it would have been more difficult to argue that social modellists, or materialists, are inextricably trapped in the biology/society, disability/impairment, dualisms. I would argue that it is quite possible simultaneously to make a conceptual distinction between impairment and disability, reconceptualize the latter as a form of social oppression, understand that bodily variations classified as impairments are materially shaped by the interaction of social and biological factors and processes, *and* appreciate that impairment is a culturally constructed category which exists in particular times and places.

Gender, and the personal (private) versus the political (public)
Postmodernism has been very influential within feminism and is widely used in deconstructing the sex/gender dichotomy, for example, in the influential work of Judith Butler (1993). By privileging the discursive construction of 'difference', postmodernism lends itself particularly well to feminist perspectives in Disability Studies (Shildrick and Price 1996; Price and Shildrick 1998; Corker 1998a; Corker and French 1999; see also Chapter 6). However, there is no single feminist view, and other disabled feminist thinkers, such as Susan Wendell, find the deconstructionist analyses of postmodernist feminism on the subject of 'the body' to be highly problematic because it assumes an 'ideal' body and is 'alienated from bodily experiences' (Wendell 1996: 168).

On the private/public and personal/political dualisms evident in Disability Studies, postmodernist feminists such as Mairian Corker take issue with the assertions of those (usually male) social modellists who argue that we should not concern ourselves with the personal experience of living with either impairment or disability (Corker and French 1999). I discussed this matter at length in Chapter 4, and do not need to repeat the debate on the question of 'the place of the personal'. The important issue here is whether, as in Corker's and others' view, the failure of influential social modellists to address the personal is inextricably bound up with their materialist approach (Corker 1998a; Corker and French 1999). I would suggest that whilst it is certainly true that (male) materialists in Disability Studies frequently reproduce the private/public and personal/political dualisms, my own approach to personal experience in this text testifies to the fact that this is not a necessary corollary of adopting a materialist perspective. Thus it is necessary to make a conceptual distinction between the failure to address the personal, and the adoption of a materialist perspective *per se*. To put it another way, in making the personal political there is common ground between feminists of different theoretical persuasions.

So once again, whilst acknowledging that those using postmodernist perspectives identify some key weaknesses in the work of influential social modellists, my argument is that that these do not necessarily derive from materialism in and of itself, but from the limited way that social modellists have utilized elements of materialism and failed to take up some of the important theoretical developments in feminism and other areas. Thus I do not agree that the solution to, or the overcoming of, these weaknesses is the exclusive prerogative of postmodernism, including feminist postmodernism. In fact they lie, in my view, in the emergence of a stronger voice for material-ist feminism in Disability Studies.

Endings: ways forward?

This chapter's discussion of historical materialist and postmodernist perspec-tives and their applications in Disability Studies has highlighted more differ-ences than similarities. Materialists have sought to explain the material foundations of disability in relations of production, have highlighted socio-structural barriers which exclude people with impairment, but have tended to downplay the role of cultural practices in disablism, matters of personal experience, impairment (except Abberley), and gender differences. Post-modernists have sought to describe the social construction of the (gendered) categories 'disabled' and 'impaired', have analysed the cultural processes of constitutive othering and the 'disciplining' of the body, but have largely ignored the real materiality of bodies and the fact that for most disabled people life is about a material struggle for existence.

Given that these theoretical perspectives cover such different ground, perhaps Disability Studies should seek a synthesis of these (and perhaps other) approaches so that all features of the socio-structural, the cultural and the experiential are addressed? Calling for syntheses has a certain 'wouldn't it be nice' appeal, but a synthesis is not an option – the philosophical, epistemological and ontological foundations of these theoretical approaches make them incompatible. This does not mean, however, that only one theor-etical perspective should be pursued at the expense of others. On the con-trary, dogma and rigid orthodoxy should be avoided at all costs. Disability Studies is enriched by accommodating a range of theoretical perspectives, and through the purposive and lively intellectual engagements between those adopting different approaches. Of course it is true that historical materialism, and Marxism generally, has had no shortage of dogmatists in its time, but the more recent postmodernist tradition, in feminism and elsewhere, is some-times equally dogmatic, uses inaccessible language, and frequently adopts an arrogant disdain for all versions of 'modernist' thought despite an avowed tolerance of 'difference' in the realm of ideas. What is required is tolerance and openness on all sides.

The value of detailed postmodernist explorations of cultural practices and discourses is to be welcomed and not at all to be denied. Despite my criticisms, I have enjoyed and learned an enormous amount from those pursuing post-modern perspectives in Disability Studies and elsewhere. The point is that, for me, these explorations of the cultural are not enough (either intellectually or politically), and I cannot agree with the exclusive emphasis on the cultural and the wholesale rejection of materialism and other 'modernist' systems of know-ledge. In particular, the apparent radicalism of postmodernism's exposure of the 'power' exercised through discursive practices based on the writings of Foucault – the disciplining power of medicine and so forth – is interesting, useful, but ultimately limited. I cannot help wanting to ask: Why do particular social groups have this power? What is its material basis? It is frequently forgotten that one does not have to be a postmodernist or a poststucturalist to appreciate that knowledge is both a 'social construct' and fundamentally bound up with the exercise of power (Murphy 1994; Craib 1997; S. Ward 1997). The discussion earlier in this chapter demonstrates that we find this appreciation in the materialist premises of Marx and Engels. In fact, sociological approaches *in general* see knowledge as a social construct (Craib 1997: 4). What really distinguishes postmodernist perspectives from other theoretical approaches is not the contention that knowledge is socially produced, and historically and culturally variable, but the deconstructionist pushing of this logic to an idealist and sceptical extreme (at least in the 'strong' forms of postmodernism) so that there is no reality independent of ideas, no materiality prior to discourses.

My own view is that a non-reductionist materialist feminism offers the best hope for understanding and explaining disability, impairment and impairment effects, and the gendered nature of these. As indicated, this means starting out with a social relational conception of disability, and seeking to explain disablism in terms of its roots in the level of development of the productive forces, the social relations of production and reproduction, and in the cultural formations and ideologies in society. In Disability Studies, an *explicitly* materialist feminist perspective is hardly discernible, although the work of Fine and Asch (1988), Jenny Morris (1991; 1995; 1996) and Susan Wendell (1996) is important and suggests some ways forward. As discussed earlier, there is nothing in the literature (to my knowledge) on the historical roots of disabled women's oppression in the particularities of production and reproduction in the capitalist epoch. There is much empirical research and theorizing to be done here.

On the question of impairment there is also much to be done from a materialist feminist perspective if there is to be a non-reductionist materialist ontology of the body. I do not accept the postmodernist view that any ideas about 'the human body' being a real, material entity, with morphological, anatomical and genetic characteristics which exist independently of 'scientific' and other discourses about the body, automatically signals a descent into a modernist ontology of the 'fixed', 'unchanging' and 'transhistorical' human body, with an accompanying categorization of bodies into 'normal' and 'impaired' types, and a belief that the biological will determine the social. It should be possible to develop a materialist perceptive on the body, on impairment, which does not collapse into fixed, categorical, universalistic and biologically determinist ways of thinking. At the same time, such a perspective can, and should, hold to the position that this material reality is always and everywhere overlaid with socially constructed ideas about the body.

Perhaps medical sociology holds some of the answers? It is to debates between Disability Studies writers and medical sociologists that I now turn.

Notes

1 This paragraph relies heavily on the published record of Sally Sainsbury's contribution to the Social and Community Planning Research (1989) seminar, 'Researching disability: methodological issues'.

2 There is a parallel between Abberley's arguments here and those found in debates about the social explanation of health inequalities – see, for example, Blane *et al.* (1996) and Benzeval *et al.* (1995). It is interesting that academics in Disability Studies and those sociologists and others involved in health inequalities research seem to occupy different universes – the two literatures hardly ever meet. Much could be gained by dialogue between the two.

3 I am influenced here by the unpublished writings of Quentin Rudland (1998). Rudland suggests a new synthesis between the most progressive aspects of neo-Darwinian evolutionary biological theory (which is thriving in the life sciences) and historical materialism (which is considered *passé* by many in the social sciences) would open up new ways of thinking, dialectically, about the changing manifestations and significance of human 'adaptations' and 'maladaptations', and the social and material contexts in which they occur.

4 Lawrence Cahoone (1996) discusses the relationship between the decline of Marxism and the rise of postmodernism in intellectual circles in the West. He notes that from the early 1970s Marxism was either profoundly reinterpreted or abandoned in the face of the widespread acknowledgement of Stalinist atrocities in the Soviet Union, the recognition that so-called 'socialism' in the Soviet Union and other 'communist' states was undesirable, and the loss of hope in a utopian socialist future: 'lacking a historical *telos* or goal, it seemed that the world had become centerless and pointless once again. Postmodernism, a wayward stepchild of Marxism, is in a sense a generation's realization that it is orphaned' (Cahoone 1996: 10). Cahoone is careful to note, however, that there is no single postmodern family, no essential commonality – there are conflicting views among postmodernists and some refuse to be known by that name.

8

Disability Studies and medical sociology

Introduction

The sociological study of chronic illness and disability (defined as restrictions of activity caused by impairment) is well established, part of the now distinct sociological subdiscipline of medical sociology, or the sociology of health and illness. Medical sociology traces its lineage to the classic writings of Parsons (1951), Mechanic (1962), Goffman (1961; 1963) and Freidson (1970). Its growth and diversification over the years has resulted in a large body of literature encompassing a variety of research methods and theoretical perspectives (Turner 1987; Gerhardt 1989; Bury 1997). Within medical sociology, the field known as the sociology of chronic illness and disability has developed apace, particularly the seam of research in the 1980s on 'the experience of illness and disability' (Anderson and Bury 1988; Conrad 1990; Bury 1991; 1997; Kelly and Field 1996). The theoretical perspectives which have most heavily shaped this 'experience of illness' work are symbolic interactionism, phenomenology and, more recently, Foucauldian postmodernism.[1]

In what ways does the younger Disability Studies differ from the sociology of chronic illness and disability? Most commentators in either field would answer, 'a great deal'. This chapter explores this question, examining areas of divergence and overlap, or potential overlap. I should declare at the start that I see myself as a writer located within both Disability Studies and medical sociology. I have learned an enormous amount from each of these literatures whilst pursuing a materialist feminist approach in both. This location is not a comfortable one because on the one hand medical sociology is usually written off as 'medical model' and thus disablist by disability activists and writers, whilst on the other hand the 'social model' of disability is strongly critiqued by some who plough their academic furrow in the sociology of chronic illness and disability. There are very significant differences in approach between Disability Studies and medical sociology, but, as I shall discuss below, there is now at least some dialogue between the two camps. This chapter is offered in the spirit of encouraging further dialogue. First, the 'divide' is outlined.

The divide

Disability Studies

In Britain, a number of academics whose work has been influential in founding Disability Studies as a distinct intellectual enterprise hinging on the social model of disability characterize their work as sociological. For example, Oliver (1990: x–xi) tells the reader:

> As a disabled sociologist, my own experience of marginalisation has been more from the sociological community than from society at large. A sociologist having either a personal or a professional interest in disability will not find disability occupies a central or even a marginal place on the sociological agenda.

He goes on to say that even in medical sociology, where at least disability is addressed, the approach taken is unhelpful: 'In recent years medical sociology has grown faster than most other areas, but within this subdivision, medical sociologists have been unable to distinguish between illness and disability and have proceeded as if they are the same thing' (Oliver 1990: xi). Disability Studies, as a sociology of disability linked to the disabled people's movement (Barton 1996b), grew up in conscious opposition to medical sociology (Barnes and Mercer 1996b). The writings of Erving Goffman (1961; 1963), so influential in medical sociological accounts of living with chronic illness and disability, have come in for particular criticism (see, for example, Finkelstein 1980; Oliver 1990; 1996c; Abberley 1993). It is argued that Goffman's interactionist focus on the micro-social consequences of the presence of stigmatized conditions in social interactions results in the representation of disabled people as passive victims of prejudice, as people who live with the unfortunate but inevitable social consequences of being impaired. In Goffman's analysis, attention is given to the way disabled individuals socially 'manage' their conditions, wherever possible by concealment strategies, so that their presentation of self in day-to-day encounters with 'normals' is minimally disruptive. In line with interpretative perspectives more generally, Goffman was interested in social meanings and individual behaviours; there is no consideration of the wider social structure and the ways in which disability might be theorized in socio-political terms.[2]

Medical sociology

Much of the research on living with particular forms of chronic illness and disability carried out by medical sociologists bears the imprint of Goffman's approach and, together with phenomenological thinking, focuses on matters of social meaning, biographical disruption, illness narratives, 'negotiated orders', and the details of individual coping, management, adjustment and adaptation – on the part of 'sufferers' and family members (see, for example, Glaser and Strauss 1965; Kleinman 1980; Bury 1982; Strauss and Glaser 1984; Fitzpatrick *et al.* 1984; Williams 1984; Anderson and Bury 1988; Kleinman 1988; *Social Science and Medicine* 1990; Radley 1993; 1994; Frank 1995; Pinder 1995; Kelly 1996).[3] As Gareth Williams (1996a: 199) states: 'The attempt to understand the meaning of experience by looking at it in context. lies at the heart of the medical sociological project', that is, experience from the point of view of the person affected. In discussing the 'meaning of illness', medical sociologists consider two things: first, the symbolic 'significance' of illness which impacts on self-identity ('what this condition means for who I am'); and second, the 'consequences' that illness has at a practical and social level for individual lives in terms of its impact on roles and activities (Bury 1997: 124). Change over time is an important theme given the progressive and/or variable nature of many chronic illnesses, and thus there is attention to illness trajectories and living with uncertainty and instability. More recently, some medical sociologists of chronic illness have been engaged with questions raised by the emergence in mainstream sociology of 'the sociology of the body' and related postmodernist perspectives (see, for example, Turner 1992; Nettleton 1995; Kelly and Field 1996; Bury 1997).

It is not my intention to review this body of medical sociological literature here – a task which has already been helpfully undertaken by some within the tradition (Conrad 1990; Bury 1991; 1997; Kelly and Field 1996). Rather, I want to focus on issues raised in the recent debate which has ensued between some Disability Studies writers and a number of medical sociologists consequent on the mutual acknowledgement that academics in these domains should talk to one another about the meaning and study of disability, and about 'the divide' between these corpora.

The debate

Events of particular significance in connection with recent dialogue are: first, the debate held at a conference entitled 'Accounting for Illness and Disability' organized in 1995 by the Disability Studies writers, Colin Barnes and Geof Mercer, specifically to explore differences between Disability Studies and the sociology of chronic illness and disability (key conference papers were later published in Barnes and Mercer 1996a); second, the exchange published in the journal *Disability and Society* between Disability Studies writers Tom Shakespeare and Nick Watson (1997) on the one hand, and Ruth Pinder (1997) whose research is located in the sociology of chronic illness on the other (these papers are brought together in Barton and Oliver 1997).

It is important to note that this debate between Disability Studies writers and medical sociologists cannot simply be reduced to a division between the disabled and the non-disabled respectively. On both sides, some writers are impaired and disabled and some are not, although most writers in Disability

Studies have personal experience of impairment and disability. In the final analysis, writers' locations are about individual biographies, personal politics and theoretical perspectives.[4] I now want to discuss, in turn, three themes or issues in the debate: conceptualizing disability; understanding experience; and disability research.

Conceptualizing disability

Medical sociologists and Disability Studies writers are at odds over the linked questions of what disability is and how it is caused (Bury 1996a; 1997; Oliver 1996a; 1996b; 1996c; Pinder 1996; 1997; Shakespeare and Watson 1997). This was examined at some length in Chapter 2 in connection with the disability definitional riddle, but it is worth revisiting the key points here.

First, the medical sociological perspective. Utilizing the International Classification of Impairments, Disabilities and Handicaps, Michael Bury defines disability as 'restrictions of activity' and sees these restrictions as caused, in the main, by chronic illness and impairment. One of the merits of the ICIDH schema, from medical sociologists' point of view, is precisely the fact that its development marked a break with a medical model perspective. Disability is no longer conceived of as the illness or impairment itself (Disability = Impairment), but as the consequential impact of illness or impairment on the activities of daily living and social interaction (Impairment → Disability). Thus, the ICIDH is seen as representing an important step forward because it considers the individual in social context. The interaction between bodies, socio-environmental contexts and milieux is then foregrounded. In one paper, Bury goes so far as to say that it is 'handicap' which is its most important element in the ICIDH/WHO schema: 'It was the emphasis on handicap which mattered most, in its attempt to point to the social disadvantage which may result from the social restrictions and conditions within which disability is experienced' (1996a: 30). However, as Gareth Williams has noted, in practice medical sociologists have given very little priority to exploring handicap: 'the work of many sociologists starts off by viewing the experience of chronic illness and disablement in its context of social and economic circumstances, but gets side-tracked into increasingly solipsistic explorations of identity and self' (Williams 1996a: 209–10). Bury's (1996a; 1997) reaction to the social model of disability is to question its assertion that disability (restrictions of activity) is caused entirely by social barriers and to argue that it expresses an 'oversocialised' and 'unidimensional' view. He also questions the credibility of this 'oppression model' on the grounds that most disabled people do not support it (that is, do not think of themselves as oppressed). Whilst he has recently conceded that, 'as has been argued, some aspects of disability are clearly a function of social expectations and the impact of social structure' (Bury 1997: 120), he nevertheless remains convinced that the social model is simplistically socially reductionist.

Turning to Disability Studies, we saw in Chapter 2 how writers such as Mike

Oliver see the ICIDH as another version of the oppressive medical model because it posits impairment/illness as the cause of impaired people's restricted activity and related disadvantage in contemporary society. Social modellists assert that these restrictions are caused by the existence of oppressive social barriers in society. However, I have pointed out that in his opposition to the medical sociology stance, Oliver (1996a; 1996b) does something problematic. He both reiterates the UPIAS social relational conceptualization of disability (as the social imposition of restrictions of activity on people with impairments) and invokes what I have called the property definition of disability (as restriction of activity). Oliver tends to conflate, or to fail to maintain a clear conceptual distinction between, a social relational formulation of disability and a property definition of disability. The result is that the UPIAS social relational definition is *extended*, so that *all* restrictions of activity experienced by people with impairment are attributed to social causes (Social Barriers → Disability).

Here, the key point about this problematic merging of a social relational and a property conceptualization of disability is that its persistence serves to fuel the medical sociology versus Disability Studies stand-off. On the one side, medical sociologists use a property definition of disability in their own work but are also able to attribute it to the social model, the result being that they see the denial of the 'disabling' effects of illness and impairment in the 'social' or 'oppression' model as somewhat absurd. On the other side, social modellists have not completely broken with a property definition of disability and tend to shift between it and a social relational understanding of disability. By not *consistently* reformulating disability as an unequal and oppressive sociopower relationship (between those socially constructed as 'impaired' (or chronically ill) and those constructed as 'normal' or unimpaired in society) social modellists let medical sociologists off the hook. The rather crude social modellist assertion that 'all restrictions of activity are caused by social barriers' can easily be dismissed by medical sociologists, and the latter are not then compelled to address seriously the question of whether or not disabled people are socially oppressed.

I shall return to this theme in the final section of the chapter, but now want to turn to the second issue of relevance in the debate: understanding experience.

Understanding experience

The keen interest which medical sociologists have in studying the personal experiences of those living with chronic illness contrasts starkly with the position of social modellists like Vic Finkelstein who argue that a focus on the personal experience of either disability or impairment is diversionary (see Chapter 4). In this book I, like some others in Disability Studies, have strongly criticized this social modellist eschewal of experience. The point to emphasize here, however, is that the issue is not simply about whether or not to pay attention to experience (discussed at length in Chapter 4), but also about why and how experience is explored and interpreted in a substantive sense. In part, this relates to research methods, discussed below, but it also concerns epistemological and ontological matters: What kind of knowledge does one hope to obtain, or give credibility to, by focusing on experience? What does the experience of illness tell us about the nature of being in the world? On these questions, medical sociologists and Disability Studies writers (that is, those who *do* examine the experience of living with disability and impairment) are a long way apart.

As discussed above, sociologists of chronic illness and disability draw inspiration from symbolic interactionism and phenomenology, and examine the illness experience within the purview of these perspectives because it enriches particular kinds of sociological understanding of what it means to be human in relation to consciousness, identity and social action. For sociologists, the empirical study of the experiences of chronically ill people (and members of their families) illuminates these particular features of 'the social'. Disability Studies writers, on the other hand, are interested in understanding disability and its forms of manifestation. The adherence to a social modellist perspective for political purposes (regardless of any personal reservations concerning the analytical strengths of this model) means that if Disability Studies writers do examine the experience of disability and impairment then this is not as an end in itself, but as a means of illustrating the ways in which discrimination and oppression operate. As stated at the beginning of Chapter 5, the interest for Disability Studies lies mainly in what the experiences of individuals with impairment can tell us about the nature of the disablism rooted in wider socio-structural and cultural contexts. To cite Liz Stanley (1993: 45) again on the sociology of auto/biography, 'from one person we can recover social processes and social structure, networks, social change and so forth, for people are located in a social and cultural environment which constructs and shapes not only *what* we see but also *how* we see it'.

As a consequence, in their empirical research, medical sociologists and Disability Studies researchers are not looking for the same things when they explore people's experiences of living with disability and impairment, and are seeking to generate different kinds of knowledge. They ask people different questions about their experiences, seeking to generate accounts or narratives about experience which have a particular emphasis. The focus is on different dimensions of the experiential, and involves searching and selecting from data with different features of the social in mind. Of course there is some overlap, but on the whole there is divergence in purpose and intent. In taking their dialogue forward, I think Disability Studies researchers and medical sociologists could usefully explore these kinds of differences in much more depth.

In both medical sociology and Disability Studies, there has been increasing use of narrative analysis, reflecting a growing interest in narratives and auto/biography in sociology and feminism more generally (Riessman 1993; Stanley 1993; Somers 1994; Plummer 1995). Once again, though, we see that medical sociologists and Disability Studies writers are looking for different types of knowledge in narratives. Narratives are the 'stories' that people tell about their lives and experiences – for example, in their own written accounts and in unstructured interviews – and narrative analyses seek to explore both the structure, content and context of these stories by treating them as integral wholes. This contrasts with traditional methods in qualitative research where experiential accounts are fragmented into pieces of data that can be used cross-sectionally in the identification of themes (Riessman 1993). In medical sociology, exploring individuals' illness narratives has been recognized as a powerful way of understanding the impact of illness on self-identity and biographical disruption, especially in connection with change over time (Williams 1984; 1996a; Radley 1993; Frank 1995). Gareth Williams has used this approach in his own research and found it of considerable value, but he also notes:

> In the end, however, the danger in much of this work is that it loses sight altogether of the structures which make the experience take the shape it does. History and even biography are dissolved in ever deeper phenomenological penetration into the interstices of self and world. What started out as a sociological analysis becomes part of a quasi-religious or spiritual quest for the truth which illness is supposed to reveal.
>
> (Williams 1996a: 202)

In Disability Studies, Tom Shakespeare has perhaps done most to advance interest in narrative research (1996a; 1997b; Shakespeare *et al.* 1996; but see also Booth 1996; Booth and Booth 1997), an approach which I have also used elsewhere (Thomas 1998a; 1998b; 1999). In Shakespeare's research with Gillespie-Sells and Davies on disabled sexuality (Shakespeare *et al.* 1996) the work of Ken Plummer (1995) on the sociology of story-telling is acknowledged as a key influence. But in contrast with medical sociologists, and as with research on experience more generally, Disability Studies writers locate individuals' narratives in the wider socio-cultural context, and explore narratives principally, though not exclusively, for what they tell us about disablism and other forms of social oppression.

A final point in this section is that the gendered nature of disability has been even less well addressed by medical sociologists than it has within Disability Studies. Medical sociologists certainly note the significance of gender and age factors in relation to the epidemiology of chronic illness (Bury 1997), but when it comes to exploring the experience of illness and disability its gendered character goes largely unexamined. What, for example, is the significance of gender difference for changes in self-identity in the face of chronic illness, the meaning of illness, disrupted biographies? In reviews of research in the field, there is frequent reference to 'sufferers', 'families and carers', and 'patients', but these individuals and groups are often strangely ungendered, unsexed, unclassed, without 'race', and ageless. Feminist perspectives are not prominent in the sociology of chronic illness tradition. In my view, matters of gender (and other social 'differences') need to be addressed more seriously in any future exchanges between Disability Studies and medical sociology on the experience of illness/impairment and disability.

Doing disability research

Emancipatory research

Within Disability Studies, there continues to be a considerable amount of discussion about the preferred form and content of disability research. Early discussions identified the need for such research to be 'emancipatory' – to adopt an 'emancipatory research paradigm' (Barnes and Mercer 1997a; see also Rioux and Bach 1994). Influential social modellists such as Mike Oliver (1992; 1997), Colin Barnes (1997b; Barnes and Mercer 1997a), Gerry Zarb (1992; 1997), and Len Barton (1996b) have argued that research on disability must aspire to be emancipatory if it is to be of any real assistance to disabled people, otherwise it will work against disabled people and shore up disablism. Researchers, they contend, have to align themselves – 'which side are you on?', 'are you for us or against us?', 'are you going to treat us as "objects" in research, exploit us for your own aggrandizement or that of your profession, or collaborate with us by ensuring that we have a (or the) key role in determining the research agenda, the research methods, and the outcomes of research?'. This stark posing of the matter is not surprising given the history of medical and most social scientific research on disability. In the way it has been conceived, organized and conducted, as well as in the nature and use of results, traditional disability research in medicine, rehabilitation, psychology, sociology and social policy has been carried out by representatives of professional groups with little or no consultation with, or involvement of, disabled people themselves (other than as research subjects). The consequence of much of this research, it is argued, is not just to alienate disabled people but to positively reinforce disablism in society.[5] With the emergence of the disabled people's movement and the development of the social model of disability, the disability research conducted *on* disabled people from the 'outside' became a focus for critique. Disability Studies sought to develop, and secure funding for, its own social modellist programme of research with its own research agenda, ethics and approved methods. Examples of funded Disability Studies research include Barnes's research on discrimination for BCODP (Barnes 1991); Zarb and Nadash's BCODP-funded research on the costs and quality of services provided by local authorities as compared with those purchased by people through direct or indirect payments (Zarb and Nadash 1994); Morris's (1993c; 1997) research on community care services and, more recently, on disabled children; the ESRC-funded research project on 'Measuring Disablement in Society' (see Zarb 1995; 1997); and the current ESRC-funded research project on 'Life as a Disabled Child'.[6]

In the introduction to their edited collection of papers, *Doing Disability Research*, Colin Barnes and Geof Mercer provide a helpful review of the debate within Disability Studies on disability research. They highlight the importance of a series of seminars on the topic funded by the Joseph Rowntree Foundation in the late 1980s and early 1990s which resulted in a national conference and a special issue of the journal *Disability, Handicap and Society* in 1992, noting that:

> [p]robably the most influential contribution was Mike Oliver's call for disability research to follow 'what has variously been called critical enquiry, praxis or emancipatory research' (1992: 107). At its heart is a political commitment to confront disability by changing: the social relations of research production, including the role of funding bodies; the relationship between researchers and those being researched; and the links between research and policy initiatives.
>
> (Barnes and Mercer 1997b: 5)

Gerry Zarb (1992; 1997) drew a distinction between emancipatory research and participatory research. In the latter, disabled people are simply involved in the research process, whereas in the former the research is 'actually controlled by them as part of a broader process of empowerment . . . The active participation of disabled people is therefore a necessary but not a sufficient condition for emancipatory research' (Zarb 1997: 51–2). He pointed out that one of the great obstacles to emancipatory research is the 'material relations of research production' which prevail, that is, the way that the funders of research exercise control over the content, process and outcome of research.[7] In very recent debate about research within Disability Studies the focus is on the difficulties (or impossibility) of actually doing emancipatory disability research (Barnes and Mercer 1997a; Oliver 1997; Zarb 1997), and on questioning its desirability (Shakespeare 1997b; 1997c). Another theme is the role and responsibility of non-disabled researchers in Disability Studies (see Stone and Priestley 1996; Priestley 1997). Thus, there are many issues left unresolved.

Business as usual and researcher independence

Unlike Disability Studies writers, sociologists of chronic illness and disability appear to be relatively content with their own research practices and methods and have not subjected these to the same kind of critical scrutiny. They see these as adequately governed by codes of professional research ethics (such as those laid down by the British Sociological Association) and by the checking mechanisms afforded by the processes of academic peer review. It is not accidental that it is in feminism, Disability Studies, and other domains of study dealing with social oppression that research paradigms and methods, and their epistemological significance, have been the subject of detailed reassessment. Researchers in these areas are acutely aware of the potential for research to constitute an oppressive practice, or to contribute to oppressive social structures and processes, and debates within feminism on these questions have been especially influential (Roberts 1981; Stanley and Wise 1983;

1993; Harding 1987; Stanley 1990; Maynard and Purvis 1994; Skeggs 1995a; see also Chapter 6). However, some medical sociologists are aware of the critiques and research challenges presented by Disability Studies. Bury, for example, has responded by strongly defending sociological research, but does note that:

> in the future it seems clear that (funded) research projects will need to take into account the political agendas of specific groups of the chronically sick and disabled more than they have in the past. The active involvement of 'client groups' in research design and conduct is rapidly growing. One benefit of the current debate is the view that medical sociologists might have held earlier, that they were providing a voice for the voiceless, will need to be more carefully considered in the future.
>
> (Bury 1997: 140)

Bury questions the Disability Studies assertion that sociological and other forms of disability research have alienated disabled people – 'this charge is not supported by any systematic empirical evidence' (Bury 1996a: 28) – and argues that some of this research, like the OPCS disability study (Martin *et al.* 1988), has had a beneficial social policy impact for disabled people (see Chapter 2). Further, social research 'has often involved challenging a number of entrenched interests, especially within medicine and government circles' (Bury 1996b: 112). He also adamantly defends the right of researchers to exercise academic freedom (as far as is possible within the many constraints on research), that is, to be 'independent', arguing that only a minority of disabled people support the social modellist perspective and that it is thoroughly undesirable to insist that researchers adhere to any one 'politically correct' perspective (Bury 1996a; 1996b; 1997; see also Barnes 1997b). Interestingly, on the question of academic freedom, Disability Studies writer Tom Shakespeare (1997b; 1997c) holds a similar position:

> is [my research] emancipatory research? To be honest I don't know and I don't really care. I am a pluralist, and would rather follow my own intellectual and ethical standards, rather than trying to conform to an orthodoxy. I don't follow recipes when I cook, and I'm not keen on following imposed rules when I research. However, I think I share the basic commitment which underlies the notion of emancipatory research, although it is for others to judge by the results.
>
> (Shakespeare 1997b: 185–6)

This characteristically forthright statement by Shakespeare is made in the context of a clearly worked-out political adherence to the social model (Shakespeare and Watson 1997) and a personal and professional set of research ethics. Perhaps – as Gareth Williams (1996a; 1996b) has argued – the American disabled sociologist and activist, Irving Zola, got it right? Williams applauds the fact that Zola was willing to examine disability from many points of view, to be pluralistic and open to the use of different research methods, whilst at the same time 'his politics [were] unwavering in the articulation of demands for independence and an end to discrimination' (Williams 1996a: 207).

Issues surrounding disability research, whilst apparently straightforward ('whose side are you on?') are thus, in practice, complex and difficult to resolve. There are no easy answers. What are the prospects for a more fruitful debate between Disability Studies and medical sociology on this and the other themes discussed?

Endings: ways forward?

In my view there is something to be gained from greater interaction, or perhaps even collaboration, between Disability Studies and medical sociology. To give just one small example from my own experience: whilst I agree with much of the social modellist critique of Erving Goffman's analysis (not surprising for a materialist) and its common usage within medical sociology, I have also found Goffman's work on the micro-social dimensions of stigma to be very insightful and informative. On a personal level it has helped me, together with social modellist writings, to come to a sociological understanding of my own behaviour in concealing impairment (see Chapter 3). Thus, it is quite possible for something positive to come of drawing on *both* social modellist and medical sociological approaches. In particular, Disability Studies could usefully learn from medical sociology in developing its capacity to research and analyse the experience of living with disability and impairment effects – *as long as* individual experience is not examined just for its own sake but is connected up with broader socio-structural and cultural structures and processes, and with a political commitment to disability rights. I have argued at length in this book for the location of experience in its broader socio-structural context, something that interactionist and phenomenological sociologists of chronic illness usually have no interest in doing. Looked at from another angle, we can see that at issue here are matters of 'structure and agency' – the old sociological conundrum. As a number of commentators in both medical sociology and Disability Studies have noted, underlying their differences in approach is the structure/agency or structure/action dualism. Medical sociologists privilege social action or agency, whilst social modellists tend to privilege structure. Disability Studies needs to find ways to overcome this dualism, or at least to encourage analyses that bridge agency and structure.

The key hurdle to collaboration, however, is medical sociologists' rejection of the 'oppression' (social) model of disability. I have argued that, in part, this rejection is bound up with the fact that social modellists lack a consistent social relational conceptualization of disability and commonly advance the easily refuted argument that all restrictions of activity experienced by people with impairment are caused by social barriers. In this book I have tried to make the case for the consistent use of a social relational perspective, and for the theoretical development of this way of thinking about disability. The question which is posed is not 'what causes this (or that) restriction of activity – social barriers or impairment?', but 'how is the oppressive social relationship which constitutes disability generated and sustained within social systems and cultural formations?'. Medical sociology has not, perhaps will not, accept such a social relational reformulation of disability – but in my view this has not been fully tested.[8]

Turning to disability research, there does at least appear to be some movement among medical sociologists when Bury (1997: 140) says 'in the future it seems clear that (funded) research projects will need to take into account the political agendas of specific groups of the chronically sick and disabled more than they have in the past'. However, there remain important differences between medical sociologists and Disability Studies writers in relation to the politics of research and the role of disability researchers. For myself, the political commitment of researchers to the disabled people's movement, to disabled people generally, and the struggle for an end to disablism is what, in the final analysis, makes disability research worth doing. A more significant shift in disability research funding in the direction of understanding disablism, discrimination, social exclusion and their effects – and how to combat these – is long overdue. But as I have argued in this book, Disability Studies should be broad enough to encompass research on all aspects of disability, including its experiential and psycho-emotional dimensions.

I shall end by briefly summarizing the essential features of the analytical framework for the study of disability which has emerged through the discussions in preceding chapters, and with the suggestion, perhaps naive, that this might be of interest and utility to medical sociologists as well as those in Disability Studies.

A social relational definition of disability

Disability is a form of social oppression involving the social imposition of restrictions of activity on people with impairments and the socially engendered undermining of their psycho-emotional well-being.

Disability and impairment effects

The lived experience of many people with impairment in society is shaped in fundamental ways by the interaction between, and the accumulative impact of, disability (or disablism) and impairment effects. However, a careful *analytical* distinction needs to be made between the consequences of disability and impairment effects. The most fruitful way forward is to develop an approach which understands disability as a form of social oppression, but which finds room for the examination of impairment effects.

Doing and being

Disability and impairment effects each have two dimensions which interact: first, factors and processes which serve to restrict activity ('doing'); and second, factors and processes which undermine psycho-emotional well-being ('being'). It is necessary to study both dimensions, giving a 2 × 2 matrix:

	Restrictions of activity	Impact on psycho-emotional well-being
Disability	✓	✓
Impairment effects	✓	✓

Notes

1 I will very briefly outline symbolic interactionism and phenomenology for the benefit of readers who may be unfamiliar with these perspectives (see Chapter 7 on postmodernism).

It is debatable whether *symbolic interactionism* amounts to a 'theory'; it is an approach to studying social action at the level of individuals and small groups which owes much to the work of sociologists at the University of Chicago during the 1920s. It is particularly associated with the work of George Herbert Mead, Herbert Blumer and Erving Goffman. Blumer formulated interactionist assumptions as follows:

> 1) Human beings act towards things on the basis of the meanings that the things have for them. 2) These meanings are the product of social interaction in human society. 3) These meanings are modified and handled through an interactive process that is used by each individual in dealing with the signs each encounters.
> (Craib 1992: 87)

Interactionists apply these assumptions in richly descriptive studies of the way individuals and groups engage with each other on a day-to-day basis in the social world, including individuals who have chronic illnesses and stigmatized impairments. Common criticisms of interactionism, which of course interactionists may reject, are that it is purely descriptive work and that it does not address features of the wider social structure (power, inequality, oppression).

Phenomenology was shaped by the philosophical writings of Edmund Husserl, published around the turn of the last century. Sociological applications of particular note are found in the work of Alfred Schutz, and Peter Berger and Thomas Luckman. Craib (1992: 98) summarizes the approach as follows:

> Phenomenology is concerned solely with the structures and workings of human consciousness, and its basic – though often implicit – presupposition is that the world we live in is created in consciousness, in our heads . . . The sociologist –

or any scientist, for that matter – is interested only in the world in so far as it is meaningful, and thus she must understand how we make it meaningful. This is achieved through setting aside what we normally assume we know and tracing the process of coming to know it. This setting aside of our knowledge is referred to sometimes as the 'phenomenological reduction', sometimes as 'bracketing', and in the more technical literature as *epoche.*

In the realm of illness and disability, phenomenologists are concerned with how illness and impairment become meaningful to us, and thus, how individuals' social worlds are constituted through meaning. Language obviously plays a key role. Phenomenology provided a philosophical background for ethnomethodology which is centrally concerned with the role of language and meaning in 'creating' individuals' social realities. The intellectual linkage between this approach and the key features of postmodernist and poststructuralist thinking is of note (see previous chapter). Language, meaning and culture are placed at the centre of social enquiry. One phenomenologist now cropping up in Disability Studies and elsewhere is Merleau-Ponty, a French philosopher whose interest was in the nature of 'lived experience'. For Merleau-Ponty, our knowledge of the world involves perception which is always incarnate, embodied – see Paterson (1998) for an application of this approach in Disability Studies.

2 For a good summary of Goffman's approach by a (sympathetic) medical sociologist, see Williams (1987).

3 As Bury points out, however, there are a few sociological studies which do examine the 'broader framework' of living with disability – for example, Mildred Blaxter's *The Meaning of Disability* (1976).

> Blaxter interviewed 100 patients during the year after discharge from a Scottish hospital, following treatment for a variety of chronic medical conditions . . . Blaxter was less interested in documenting the detail of interactional difficulties than in establishing the various 'problems' patients and their families faced during the year in question. These ranged from continuing medical troubles and problems with housing to wider social difficulties.
>
> (Bury 1997: 122)

4 An interesting example lending support to this point is furnished by the recent debate about disability in another academic discipline, geography. On the side of a traditional socio-medical conceptualization of disability is a self-identified visually impaired geographer, Golledge (1993; 1996), whilst on the side of radical social modellist disability politics is a self-declared non-disabled geographer, Brendan Gleeson (1996) (for more in this debate, see also Butler 1994; Imrie 1996b).

5 As discussed in Chapter 2, social modellists include in this the OPCS disability research which used the ICIDH (Abberley 1992). For interesting early debates within psychology in the USA on this question, see: Asch (1984), Asch and Fine (1988), Fine and Asch (1988).

6 It is very significant that the ESRC and other key research agencies have begun to fund Disability Studies research. In an interesting account of significant shifts in funding criteria for disability research operationalized by the Joseph Rowntree Foundation – the 'largest single independent funder of applied research and development projects in the fields of housing, social care and disability in the UK' (L. Ward 1997: 32–3) – Linda Ward states:

> there is the avowed commitment to only funding research which locates itself within the social model of disability, a policy deriving from the inception of the

Foundation's Advisory Group on Disability of which [Mike] Oliver was an original, key, member, and significant resource and ally to the author. Nowadays, an avowed commitment to the social model of disability is relatively commonplace (in principle if not in practice) but in 1988 [this] was far from true. As a major funding body, the Foundation was able to play a significant consciousness-raising role in firmly stating its commitment to the social model of disability and its expectation that those seeking funding would follow suit.

(L. Ward 1997: 34)

Another indicator of the growing influence of Disability Studies in Britain was the strength of the 'disability stream' at the 1998 British Sociological Association Annual Conference on 'The Sociology of the Body'.

7 In the UK the major funders in the disability field are: the Medical Research Council; the Department of Health, especially through the National Health Service research and development programme on 'Physical and Complex Disabilities'; the ESRC; and independent charitable funding agencies such as the Joseph Rowntree Foundation.

8 I noted earlier in this chapter that one of Bury's (1996a; 1997) objections to the 'oppression model' is that most disabled people do not support a social modellist perspective (that is, do not think of themselves as oppressed). However, the theoretical conceptualization of disabled people as socially oppressed does not stand or fall on the grounds that 'most disabled people do not see themselves as oppressed' – any more than it does in the case of women's oppression.

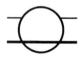

References

Abberley, P. (1987) The concept of oppression and the development of a social theory of disability, *Disability, Handicap and Society*, 2: 5–20.

Abberley, P. (1992) Counting us out: a discussion of the OPCS disability surveys, *Disability, Handicap and Society*, 7(2): 139–55.

Abberley, P. (1993) Disabled people and 'normality', in J. Swain, V. Finkelstein, S. French and M. Oliver (eds) *Disabling Barriers – Enabling Environments*. London: Sage.

Abberley, P. (1996) Work, utopia and impairment, in L. Barton (ed.) *Disability and Society: Emerging Issues and Insights*. Harlow: Longman.

Abberley, P. (1997) The limits of classical social theory in the analysis and transformation of disablement (Can this really be the end; to be stuck inside of Mobile with the Memphis Blues again?), in L. Barton and M. Oliver (eds) *Disability Studies: Past, Present and Future*. Leeds: The Disability Press.

Albrecht, G. (1992) *The Disability Business*. London: Sage.

Anderson, R. and Bury, M. (eds) (1988) *Living with Chronic Illness: The Experience of Patients and Their Families*. London: Unwin Hyman.

Appleby, Y. (1994) Out in the margins, *Disability and Society*, 9(1): 19–32.

Asch, A. (1984) The experience of disability: a challenge for psychology, *American Psychologist*, 39(5): 529–36.

Asch, A. and Fine, M. (eds) (1988) Moving disability beyond stigma, *Journal of Social Issues*, Special Issue, 44(1): 3–21.

Barnes, C. (1991) *Disabled People in Britain and Discrimination*. London: Hurst & Co.

Barnes, C. (1996) Theories of disability and the origins of the oppression of disabled people in Western society, in L. Barton (ed.) *Disability and Society: Emerging Issues and Insights*. Harlow: Longman.

Barnes, C. (1997a) A legacy of oppression: a history of disability in Western culture, in L. Barton and M. Oliver (eds) *Disability Studies: Past, Present and Future*. Leeds: The Disability Press.

Barnes, C. (1997b) Disability and the myth of the independent researcher, in L. Barton and M. Oliver (eds) *Disability Studies: Past, Present and Future*. Leeds: The Disability Press.

Barnes, C. and Mercer, G. (eds) (1996a) *Exploring the Divide: Illness and Disability*. Leeds: The Disability Press.

Barnes, C. and Mercer, G. (1996b) Introduction, in C. Barnes and G. Mercer (eds) *Exploring the Divide: Illness and Disability*. Leeds: The Disability Press.

Barnes, C. and Mercer, G. (eds) (1997a) *Doing Disability Research*. Leeds: The Disability Press.

Barnes, C. and Mercer, G. (1997b) Breaking the mould? An introduction to doing disability research, in C. Barnes and G. Mercer (eds) *Doing Disability Research*. Leeds: The Disability Press.

Barton, L. (ed.) (1996a) *Disability and Society: Emerging Issues and Insights*. Harlow: Longman.

Barton, L. (1996b) Sociology and disability: some emerging issues, in L. Barton (ed.) *Disability and Society: Emerging Issues and Insights*. Harlow: Longman.

Barton, L. and Oliver, M. (eds) (1997) *Disability Studies: Past, Present and Future*. Leeds: The Disability Press.

Begum, N. (1992) Disabled women and the feminist agenda, *Feminist Review*, 40: 70–84.

Begum, N., Hill, M. and Stevens, A. (eds) (1994) *Reflections: The Views of Black Disabled People on Their Lives and Community Care*. London: Central Council for Education and Training in Social Work.

Bendelow, G. (1993) Pain perceptions, emotions and gender, *Sociology of Health and Illness*, 15(2): 273–94.

Bendelow, G. and Williams, S.J. (1995) Transcending the dualisms: towards a sociology of pain, *Sociology of Health and Illness*, 17(2): 139–65.

Bendelow, G. and Williams, S.J. (eds) (1998) *Emotions in Social Life: Critical Themes and Contemporary Issues*. London: Routledge.

Benzeval, M., Judge, K. and Whitehead, M. (eds) (1995) *Tackling Inequalities in Health: An Agenda for Action*. London: King's Fund.

Berwick, L. (1990) *Inner Vision*. London: Arthur James.

Blane, D., Brunner, E. and Wilkinson, R. (eds) (1996) *Health and Social Organization*. London: Routledge.

Blaxter, M. (1976) *The Meaning of Disability*. London: Heinemann.

Booth, T. (1996) Sounds of still voices: issues in the use of narrative methods with people who have learning difficulties, in L. Barton (ed.) *Disability and Society: Emerging Issues and Insights*. Harlow: Longman.

Booth, T. and Booth, W. (1997) Making connections: a narrative study of adult children of parents with learning difficulties, in C. Barnes and G. Mercer (eds) *Doing Disability Research*. Leeds: The Disability Press.

Bordo, S. (1990) Feminism, postmodernism, and gender-scepticism, in L.J. Nicholson (ed.) *Feminism and Postmodernism*. London: Routledge.

Browne, S.E., Connors, D. and Stern, N. (eds) (1985) *With the Power of Each Breath: a Disabled Women's Anthology*. Pittsburgh: Cleis Press.

Bruce, I., McKennel, A. and Walker, E. (1991) *Blind and Partially Sighted People in Great Britain*. London: HMSO.

Bury, M. (1982) Chronic illness as biographical disruption, *Sociology of Health and Illness*, 4(2): 167–82.

Bury, M. (1991) The sociology of chronic illness: a review of research and prospects, *Sociology of Health and Illness*, 13(4), 451–68.

Bury, M. (1996a) Defining and researching disability: challenges and responses, in C. Barnes and G. Mercer (eds) *Exploring the Divide: Illness and Disability*. Leeds: The Disability Press.

Bury, M. (1996b) Disability and the myth of the independent researcher: a reply, *Disability and Society*, 11(1): 111–13.

Bury, M. (1997) *Health and Illness in a Changing Society*. London: Routledge.

Butler, J. (1993) *Bodies that Matter: On the Discursive Limits of 'Sex'*. London: Routledge.

Butler, R.E. (1994) Geography and vision-impaired and blind populations, *Transactions of the Institute of British Geographers*, 19(3): 366–8.

Cahoone, L. (ed.) (1996) *From Modernism to Postmodernism: An Anthology*. Oxford: Blackwell.

Campbell, J. (1997) 'Growing pains' disability politics – the journey explained, in L. Barton and M. Oliver (eds) *Disability Studies: Past, Present and Future*. Leeds: The Disability Press.

Campbell, J. and Oliver, M. (1996) *Disability Politics: Understanding Our Past, Changing Our Future*. London: Routledge.

Campling, J. (ed.) (1981) *Images of Ourselves: Women with Disabilities Talking*. London: Routledge and Kegan Paul.

Carby, H. (1982) Black feminism and the boundaries of sisterhood, in Birmingham University Centre for Contemporary Cultural Studies *The Empire Strikes Back: Race and Racism in 70s Britain*. London: Hutchinson.

Conrad, P. (1990) Qualitative research on chronic illness: a commentary on method and conceptual development, *Social Science and Medicine*, 30(11): 1257–63.

Coote, A. and Campbell, B. (1982) *Sweet Freedom: The Struggle for Women's Liberation*. London: Picador.

Corbett, J. (1994) A proud label: exploring the relationship between disability politics and gay pride, *Disability and Society*, 9(3): 343–57.

Corbett, J. (1996) *Bad-Mouthing: The Language of Special Needs*. London: Falmer.

Corker, M. (1993) Integration and deaf people: the policy and power of enabling environments, in J. Swain, V. Finkelstein, S. French and M. Oliver (eds) *Disabling Barriers – Enabling Environments*. London: Sage.

Corker, M. (1996) *Deaf Transitions*. London: Jessica Kingsley.

Corker, M. (1997) Deaf people and interpreting – the struggle in language, *Deaf Worlds*, 13(3): 13–20.

Corker, M. (1998a) *Deaf and Disabled, or Deafness Disabled?* Buckingham: Open University Press.

Corker, M. (1998b) Disability discourse in a postmodern world, in T. Shakespeare (ed.) *Disability Studies Reader*. London: Cassell.

Corker, M. and French, S. (eds) (1999) *Disability Discourse*. Buckingham: Open University Press.

Craib, I. (1992) *Modern Social Theory: From Parsons to Habermas*, 2nd edn. Hemel Hempstead: Harvester Wheatsheaf.

Craib, I. (1997) Social constructionism as a social psychosis, *Sociology*, 31(1): 1–15.

Crow, L. (1996) Including all of our lives: renewing the social model of disability, in C. Barnes and G. Mercer (eds) *Exploring the Divide: Illness and Disability*. Leeds: The Disability Press.

Davis, L.J. (ed.) (1997) *The Disability Studies Reader*. London: Routledge.

Deegan, M.J. and Brooks, N. (eds) (1985) *Women and Disability*. New Brunswick, NJ: Transaction Books.

Disability Alliance Educational and Research Association (1995) *Disability Rights Handbook, April 1995–April 1996*, 20th edn. London: Disability Alliance Educational and Research Association.

DPI (1982) Proceedings of the First World Congress, Singapore: Disabled People's International.

Driedger, D. and Gray, S. (eds) (1992) *Imprinting Our Image: An International Anthology by Women with Disabilities*. Charlottetown, Prince Edward Island: Gynergy Books.

Dyer, R. (1997) *White*. London: Routledge.

Engels, F. (1972) *The Origin of the Family, Private Property and the State*. London: Lawrence and Wishart.

Evans, M. (1993) Reading lives: how the personal might be social, *Sociology*, 27(1): 5–13.

Finch, J. (1990) The politics of community care in Britain, in C. Ungerson (ed.) *Gender and Caring: Work and Welfare in Britain and Scandinavia*. Hemel Hempstead: Harvester Wheatsheaf.

Finch, J. and Groves, D. (eds) (1983) *A Labour of Love: Women, Work and Caring*. London: Routledge & Kegan Paul.

Fine, M. and Asch, A. (eds) (1988) *Women with Disabilities: Essays in Psychology, Culture and Politics*. Philadelphia: Temple University Press.

Finger, A. (1990) *Past Due: A Story of Disability, Pregnancy and Birth*. London: The Women's Press.

Finkelstein, V. (1980) *Attitudes and Disabled People: Issues for Discussion*. New York: World Rehabilitation Fund.

Finkelstein, V. (1996) Outside, 'inside out', *Coalition*, April, 30–6.

Finkelstein, V. and French, S. (1993) Towards a psychology of disability, in J. Swain, V. Finkelstein, S. French and M. Oliver (eds) *Disabling Barriers – Enabling Environments*. London: Sage.

Fitzpatrick, R., Hinton, J., Newman, S., Scambler, G. and Thomson, J. (1984) *The Experience of Illness*. London: Tavistock.

Foucault, M. (1967) *Madness and Civilisation*. London: Tavistock.

Foucault, M. (1972) *The Archaeology of Knowledge*. London: Tavistock.

Foucault, M (1973) *The Birth of the Clinic*. London: Tavistock.

Foucault, M. (1977) *Discipline and Punish*. London: Allen Lane.

Foucault, M. (1979) *The History of Sexuality*, Vol. 1, An introduction. London: Allen Lane.

Foucault, M. (1980) *Power/Knowledge* (ed. C. Gordon). Brighton: Harvester Press.

Foucault, M. (1986) *The History of Sexuality*, Vol. 2, The use of pleasure. London: Viking.

Foucault, M. (1988) *The History of Sexuality*, Vol. 3, The care of the self. London: Allen Lane.

Frank, A.W. (1991) For a sociology of the body: an analytical review, in M. Featherstone, M. Hepworth and B.S. Turner (eds) *The Body: Social Process and Cultural Theory*. London: Sage.

Frank, A.W. (1995) *The Wounded Storyteller: Body, Illness, and Ethics*. Chicago and London: University of Chicago Press.

Freidson, E. (1970) *The Profession of Medicine*. New York: Dodd-Mead.

French, S. (1993) Disability, impairment or something in between?, in J. Swain, V. Finkelstein, S. French and M. Oliver (eds) *Disabling Barriers – Enabling Environments*. London: Sage.

French, S. (1994) *On Equal Terms: Working with Disabled People*. Oxford: Butterworth-Heinemann.

Fuss, D. (1989) *Essentially Speaking: Feminism, Nature and Difference*. London: Routledge.

Garland-Thomson, R. (1994) Redrawing the boundaries of feminist disability studies, *Feminist Studies*, 20(3): 583–95.

Gerhardt, U. (1989) *Ideas about Illness: An Intellectual and Political History of Medical Sociology*. London: Macmillan.

Giddens, A. (1991) *Modernity and Self-Identity*. Cambridge: Polity Press.

Glaser, B.G. and Strauss, A.L. (1965) *Awareness of Dying*. Chicago: Aldine.

Gleeson, B.J. (1993) Second nature? The socio-spatial production of disability. Unpublished PhD thesis, Department of Geography, University of Melbourne, Australia.

Gleeson, B.J. (1996) A geography for disabled people? *Transactions of the Institute of British Geographers,* NS 21: 387–96.

Gleeson, B.J. (1997a) Disability Studies: a historical materialist view, *Disability and Society,* 12(2): 179–202.

Goffman, E. (1961) *Asylums.* New York: Doubleday.

Goffman, E. (1963) *Stigma: Some Notes on the Management of Spoiled Identity.* Harmondsworth: Penguin.

Golledge, R. (1993) Geography and the disabled: a survey with special reference to vision impaired and blind populations, *Transactions of the Institute of British Geographers,* 18(1): 63–85.

Golledge, R. (1996) Response to Gleeson and Imrie, *Transactions of the Institute of British Geographers,* NS 21: 404–11.

Graham, H. (1991) The concept of caring in feminist research: the case of domestic service, *Sociology,* 25 (1): 67–78.

Griffiths, M. (1995) *Feminisms and the Self: The Web of Identity.* London: Routledge.

Hannaford, S. (1985) *Living Outside Inside: a disabled woman's experience – towards a social and political perspective.* Berkeley, CA: Canterbury Press.

Haraway, D. (1991) *Simians, Cyborgs, and Women: the Reinvention of Nature.* London: Free Association Books.

Harding, S. (1987) *Feminism and Methodology.* Milton Keynes: Open University Press.

Harding, S. (1991) *Whose Science, Whose Knowledge? Thinking from Women's Lives.* Buckingham: Open University Press.

Harris, A., Cox, E. and Smith, C. (1971a) *Handicapped and Impaired in Great Britain,* Vol. 1. London: HMSO.

Harris, A., Cox, E. and Smith, C. (1971b) *Handicapped and Impaired in Great Britain, Economic Dimensions.* London: HMSO.

Harris, J. (1995) *The Cultural Meaning of Deafness.* Aldershot: Avebury.

Hevey, D. (1992) *The Creatures Time Forgot.* London: Routledge.

Hill Collins, P. (1990) *Black Feminist Thought: Knowledge, Consciousness, and the Politics of Empowerment.* London: Routledge.

Hillyer, B. (1993) *Feminism and Disability.* Norman and London: University of Oklahoma Press.

Hughes, B. and Paterson, K (1997) The social model of disability and the disappearing body: towards a sociology of impairment, *Disability and Society,* 12(3): 325–40.

Hunt, P. (1966) *Stigma: The Experience of Disability.* London: Geoffrey Chapman.

Imrie, R. (1996a) *Disability and the City: International Perspectives.* London: Paul Chapman.

Imrie, R. (1996b) Ableist geographies, disablist spaces: towards a reconstruction of Golledge's 'Geography and the Disabled', *Transactions of the Institute of British Geographers,* NS 21: 397–403.

Keith, L. (1992) Who cares wins? Women, caring and disability, *Disability, Handicap and Society,* 7(2): 167–75.

Keith, L. (ed.) (1994) *Mustn't Grumble: Writing by Disabled Women.* London: The Women's Press.

Kelly, M. (1996) Negative attributes of self: radical surgery and the inner and outer life-world, in C. Barnes and G. Mercer (eds) *Exploring the Divide: Illness and Disability.* Leeds: The Disability Press.

Kelly, M. and Field, D. (1996) Medical sociology, chronic illness and the body, *Sociology of Health and Illness,* 18(2): 241–57.

Kennedy, M. (1996) Sexual abuse and disabled children, in J. Morris (ed.) *Encounters with Strangers: Feminism and Disability.* London: The Women's Press.

Kleinman, A. (1980) *Patients and Healers in the Context of Culture*. London: University of California Press.

Kleinman, A. (1988) *The Illness Narratives: Suffering, Healing and the Human Condition*. New York: Basic Books.

Lechte, J. (1994) *Fifty Contemporary Thinkers: From Structuralism to Postmodernity*. London: Routledge.

Lloyd, M. (1992) Does she boil eggs? Towards a feminist model of disability, *Disability, Handicap and Society*, 7(3): 207–21.

Lonsdale, S. (1990) *Women and Disability*. London: Macmillan.

Lyotard, J.-F. (1984) *The Postmodern Condition: A Report on Knowledge*. Minneapolis: University of Minnesota Press.

Marris, V. (1996) *Lives Worth Living: Women's Experience of Chronic Illness*. London: HarperCollins.

Martin, J., Meltzer, H. and Elliot, D. (1988) *OPCS Surveys of Disability in Great Britain: Report 1 – The Prevalence of Disability among Adults*. London: HMSO.

Marx, K. (1972) *The Eighteenth Brumaire of Louis Bonaparte*. Moscow: Progress Publishers.

Marx, K. (1977) *A Contribution to the Critique of Political Economy*. Moscow: Progress Publishers.

Marx, K. and Engels, F. (1970) The German ideology, in C.J. Arthur (ed.) *The German Ideology: Student's Edition*. London: Lawrence and Wishart.

Mason, M. (1992) A nineteen-parent family, in J. Morris (ed.) *Alone Together: Voices of Single Mothers*. London: The Women's Press.

Matthews, G.W. (ed.) (1983) *Voices from the Shadows: Women with Disabilities Speak Out*. Ontario, Canada: Women's Educational Press.

Maynard, M. and Purvis, J. (eds) (1994) *Researching Women's Lives from a Feminist Perspective*. London: Taylor and Francis.

McNamara, J. (1996) Out of order: madness is a feminist and a disability issue, in J. Morris (ed.) *Encounters with Strangers: Feminism and Disability*. London: The Women's Press.

Mechanic, D. (1962) The concept of illness behaviour, *Journal of Chronic Disease*, 15: 53–63.

Miller, N. (1991) *Getting Personal: Feminist Occasions and Other Autobiographical Acts*. London: Routledge.

Morris, J. (1989) *Able Lives: Women's Experience of Paralysis*. London: The Women's Press.

Morris, J. (1991) *Pride Against Prejudice: Transforming Attitudes to Disability*. London: The Women's Press.

Morris, J. (ed.) (1992a) *Alone Together: Voices of Single Mothers*. London: The Women's Press.

Morris, J. (1992b) Personal and political: a feminist perspective on researching physical disability, *Disability, Handicap and Society*, 7(2): 157–66.

Morris, J. (1993a) Feminism and disability, *Feminist Review*, 43(Spring): 57–70.

Morris, J. (1993b) Gender and disability, in J. Swain, V. Finkelstein, S. French and M. Oliver (eds) *Disabling Barriers – Enabling Environments*. London: Sage.

Morris, J.(1993c) *Independent Lives? Community Care and Disabled People*. London: Macmillan.

Morris, J. (1995) Creating a space for absent voices: disabled women's experience of receiving assistance with daily living activities, *Feminist Review*, 51(Autumn): 68–93.

Morris, J. (ed.) (1996) *Encounters with Strangers: Feminism and Disability*. London: The Women's Press.

Morris. J, (1997) Gone missing? Disabled children living away from their families, *Disability and Society*, 12(2): 241–58.

Murphy, R. (1994) The sociological construction of science without nature, *Sociology*, 28(4): 957–74.

Nettleton, S. (1995) *The Sociology of Health and Illness*. Cambridge: Polity Press.

Oliver, M. (1990) *The Politics of Disablement*. London: Macmillan.

Oliver, M. (1992) Changing the social relations of research production? *Disability, Handicap and Society*, 7(2): 101–14.

Oliver, M. (1996a) Defining impairment and disability: issues at stake, in C. Barnes and G. Mercer (eds) *Exploring the Divide: Illness and Disability*. Leeds: The Disability Press.

Oliver, M. (1996b) *Understanding Disability*. London: Macmillan.

Oliver, M. (1996c) A sociology of disability or a disablist sociology?, in L. Barton (ed.) *Disability and Society: Emerging Issues and Insights*. Harlow: Longman.

Oliver, M. (1997) Emancipatory research: realistic goal or impossible dream?, in C. Barnes and G. Mercer (eds) *Doing Disability Research*. Leeds: The Disability Press.

Oliver, M., Zarb, G., Silver, J., Moore, M. and Salisbury, V. (1988) *Walking into Darkness: The Experience of Spinal Injury*. London: Macmillan.

Parsons, T. (1951) *The Social System*. New York: Free Press.

Paterson, K. (1998) Disability studies and phenomenology: finding a space for both the carnal and the political. Paper presented to the British Sociological Association Conference, Edinburgh, April.

Pinder, R. (1995) Bringing back the body without the blame? The experience of ill and disabled people at work, *Sociology of Health and Illness*, 17(5): 605–31.

Pinder, R. (1996) Sick-but-fit or fit-but-sick? Ambiguity and identity at the workplace, in C. Barnes and G. Mercer (eds) *Exploring the Divide: Illness and Disability*. Leeds: The Disability Press.

Pinder, R. (1997) A reply to Tom Shakespeare and Nicholas Watson, in L. Barton and M. Oliver (eds) *Disability Studies: Past, Present and Future*. Leeds: The Disability Press.

Plummer, K. (1995) *Telling Sexual Stories: Power, Change and Social Worlds*. London: Routledge.

Potts, T. and Price, J. (1995) Out of the blood and spirit of our lives: the place of the body in academic feminism, in L. Morley and V. Walsh (eds) *Feminist Academics: Creative Agents for Change*. London: Taylor and Francis.

Price, J. (1996) The marginal politics of our bodies? Women's health, the disability movement, and power, in B. Humphries (ed.) *Critical Perspectives on Empowerment*. Birmingham: Venture Press. (Quotations are from the original version of this paper (1995)).

Price, J. and Shildrick, M. (1998) Uncertain thoughts on the dis/abled body, in M. Shildrick and J. Price (eds) *Vital Signs: Feminist Reconfigurations of the Biological Body*. Edinburgh: Edinburgh University Press.

Priestley, M. (1995) Commonality and difference in the movement, *Disability and Society*, 10: 157–69.

Priestley, M. (1997) Who's research? A personal audit, in C. Barnes and G. Mercer (eds) *Doing Disability Research*. Leeds: The Disability Press.

Priestley, M. (1998) Constructions and creations: idealism, materialism and disability theory, *Disability and Society*, 13(1): 75–94.

Probyn, E. (1993) *Sexing the Self: Gendered Positions in Cultural Studies*. London: Routledge.

Radley, A. (ed.) (1993) *Worlds of Illness: Biographical and Cultural Perspectives on Health and Disease*. London: Routledge.

Radley, A. (ed.) (1994) *Making Sense of Illness*. London: Sage.

Riddell, S. (1996) Theorising special educational needs in a changing political climate, in L. Barton (ed.) *Disability and Society: Emerging Issues and Insights*. Harlow: Longman.

Riessman, C.K. (1993) *Narrative Analysis*. London: Sage.

Rioux, M. and Bach, M. (eds) (1994) *Disability Is Not Measles. New Research Paradigms in Disability*. New York, Ontario: Roeher Institute.

Roberts, H. (ed.) (1981) *Doing Feminist Research*. London: Routledge & Kegan Paul.

Robinson, C. and Stalker, K. (eds) (1998) *Growing Up with Disability*. London: Jessica Kingsley.

Rowbotham, S. (1972) *Women, Resistance and Revolution*. Harmondsworth: Penguin.

Rudland, Q. (1998) Darwinism, Marxism and disability. Unpublished paper.

Safilios-Rothschild, C. (1970) *The Sociology and Social Psychology of Disability and Rehabilitation*. New York: Random House.

Saxton, M. and Howe, F. (eds) (1987) *With Wings: An Anthology of Literature by and about Women with Disabilities*. New York: The Feminist Press at the City University of New York.

Scheer, J. and Groce, N. (1988) Impairment as a human constant: cross-cultural and historical perspectives on variation, *Journal of Social Issues*, 44(1): 23–38.

Shakespeare, T. (1993) Disabled people's self-organisation: a new social movement? *Disability, Handicap and Society*, 8(3): 249–63.

Shakespeare, T. (1996a) Disability, identity, difference, in C. Barnes and G. Mercer (eds) *Exploring the Divide: Illness and Disability*. Leeds: The Disability Press.

Shakespeare, T. (1996b) Power and prejudice: issues of gender, sexuality and disability, in L. Barton (ed.) *Disability and Society: Emerging Issues and Insights*. Harlow: Longman.

Shakespeare, T. (1997a) Cultural representation of disabled people: dustbins of disavowal?, in L. Barton and M. Oliver (eds) *Disability Studies: Past, Present and Future*. Leeds: The Disability Press.

Shakespeare, T. (1997b) Researching disabled sexuality, in C. Barnes and G. Mercer (eds) *Doing Disability Research*. Leeds: The Disability Press.

Shakespeare, T. (1997c) Rules of engagement: changing disability research, in L. Barton and M. Oliver (eds) *Disability Studies: Past, Present and Future*. Leeds: The Disability Press.

Shakespeare, T. and Watson, N. (1997) Defending the social model, in L. Barton and M. Oliver (eds) *Disability Studies: Past, Present and Future*. Leeds: The Disability Press.

Shakespeare, T., Gillespie-Sells, K. and Davies, D. (1996) *The Sexual Politics of Disability: Untold Desires*. London: Cassell.

Shildrick, M. (1997) *Leaky Bodies and Boundaries: Feminism, Postmodernism and Bioethics*. London: Routledge.

Shildrick, M. and Price, J. (1996) Breaking the boundaries of the broken body, *Body and Society*, 2(4): 93–113.

Skeggs, B. (ed.) (1995a) *Feminist Cultural Theory: Process and Production*. Manchester: Manchester University Press.

Skeggs, B. (1995b) Introduction, in B. Skeggs (ed.) *Feminist Cultural Theory: Process and Production*. Manchester: Manchester University Press.

Skeggs, B. (1995c) Theorising, ethics and representation in feminist ethnography, in B. Skeggs (ed.) *Feminist Cultural Theory: Process and Production*. Manchester: Manchester University Press.

Skeggs, B. (1997) *Formations of Class and Gender*. London: Sage.

Social and Community Planning Research (1989) Researching disability: methodological issues, *Survey Methods Newsletter*. London: SCPR.

Social Science and Medicine (1990) Special Issue, *Social Science and Medicine*, 30(11).

Sociology (1993) Special Issue: Auto/biography, *Sociology*, 27(1).

Somers, M. (1994) The narrative construction of identity: a relational and network approach, *Theory and Society*, 23: 605–49.

Somers, M. and Gibson, G. (1994) Reclaiming the epistemological 'other': narrative and the social constitution of identity, in C. Calhoun (ed.) *Social Theory and the Politics of Identity*. Cambridge, MA: Blackwell.

Stacey, J. (1995) The lost audience: methodology, cinema history and feminist film criticism, in B. Skeggs (ed.) *Feminist Cultural Theory: Process and Production*. Manchester: Manchester University Press.

Stacey, J. (1997) Feminist theory: capital F, capital T, in V. Robinson and D. Richardson (eds) *Introducing Women's Studies*, 2nd edn. London: Macmillan.

Stanley, L. (ed.) (1990) *Feminist Praxis: Research, Theory and Espistemology in Feminist Research*. London: Routledge.

Stanley, L. (1993) On auto/biography in sociology, *Sociology*, 27(1): 41–52.

Stanley, L. (1996) The mother of invention: necessity, writing and representation, in S. Wilkinson and C. Kitzinger (eds) *Representing the Other: A Feminism and Psychology Reader*. London: Sage.

Stanley, L. and Wise, S. (1983) *Breaking Out: Feminist Consciousness and Feminist Research*. London: Routledge & Kegan Paul.

Stanley, L. and Wise, S. (1990) Method, methodology and epistemology in feminist research processes, in L. Stanley (ed.) *Feminist Praxis: Research, Theory and Espistemology in Feminist Research*. London: Routledge.

Stanley, L. and Wise, S. (1993) *Breaking Out Again*. London: Routledge.

Stewart, H., Percival, B. and Apperley, E. (eds) (1992) *The More We Get Together: Women and Disability*. Charlottetown, PEI: Gynergy Books.

Stone, E. and Priestley, M. (1996) Parasites, pawns and partners: disability research and the role of non-disabled researchers, *British Journal of Sociology*, 47(4): 699–716.

Strauss, A. and Glaser, B. (1984) *Chronic Illness and the Quality of Life*, 2nd edn. St Louis, MO: Mosby.

Stuart, O. (1993) Double oppression: an appropriate starting-point?, in J. Swain, V. Finkelstein, S. French and M. Oliver (eds) *Disabling Barriers – Enabling Environments*. London: Sage.

Swain, J., Finkelstein, V., French, S. and Oliver, M. (eds) (1993) *Disabling Barriers – Enabling Environments*. London: Sage.

Thomas, C. (1993) Deconstructing concepts of care, *Sociology*, 27(4): 649–69.

Thomas, C. (1996) Domestic labour and health: bringing it all back home, *Sociology of Health and Illness*, 17(3): 328–52.

Thomas, C. (1997) The baby and the bathwater: disabled women and motherhood in social context, *Sociology of Health and Illness*, 19(5): 622–43.

Thomas, C. (1998a) Becoming a mother: disabled women (can) do it too, *MIDIRS Midwifery Digest*, 8(3): 275–8.

Thomas, C. (1998b) Parents and family: disabled women's stories about their childhood experiences, in C. Robinson and K. Stalker (eds) *Growing Up with Disability*. London: Jessica Kingsley.

Thomas, C. (1999) Narrative identity and the disabled self, in M. Corker and S. French (eds) *Disability Discourse*. Buckingham: Open University Press.

Thomas, C. and Curtis, P. (1997) Having a baby: some disabled women's reproductive experiences, *Midwifery*, 13: 202–9.

Tolmach-Lakoff, R. (1989) Women and disability. Review essay, *Feminist Studies*, 15(2): 365–75.

Topliss, E. (1979) *Provision for the Disabled,* 2nd edn. Oxford: Blackwell and Martin Robertson.

Turner, B.S. (1987) *Medical Power and Social Knowledge.* London: Sage.

Turner, B.S. (1992) *Regulating Bodies: Essays in Medical Sociology.* London: Routledge.

United Nations (1983) *World Programme of Action Concerning Disabled Persons.* New York: United Nations.

UPIAS (1976) *Fundamental Principles of Disability.* London: Union of the Physically Impaired Against Segregation.

Verbrugge, L.M. (1995) New thinking and science on disability in mid and late life, *European Journal of Public Health,* 5(1): 20–8.

Vernon, A. (1996) A stranger in many camps: the experience of disabled black and ethnic minority women, in J. Morris (ed.) *Encounters with Strangers: Feminism and Disability.* London: The Women's Press.

Vernon, A. (1997) Fighting two different battles: unity is preferable to enmity, in L. Barton and M. Oliver (eds) *Disability Studies: Past, Present and Future.* Leeds: The Disability Press.

Walby, S. (1990) *Theorising Patriarchy.* Oxford: Blackwell.

Walby, S. (1997) *Gender Transformations.* London: Routledge.

Ward, L. (1997) Funding for change: translating emancipatory disability research from theory to practice, in C. Barnes and G. Mercer (eds) *Doing Disability Research.* Leeds: The Disability Press.

Ward, S. (1997) Being objective about objectivity: the ironies of standpoint epistemological critiques of science, *Sociology,* 31(4): 773–91.

Warmsley, J. (1997) Including people with learning difficulties: theory and practice, in L. Barton and M. Oliver (eds) *Disability Studies: Past, Present and Future.* Leeds: The Disability Press.

Wendell, S. (1989) Towards a feminist theory of disability, *Hypatia,* 4(Summer): 104–24.

Wendell, S. (1996) *The Rejected Body. Feminist Philosophical Reflections on Disability.* London: Routledge.

Williams, G. (1984) The genesis of chronic illness: narrative reconstruction, *Sociology of Health and Illness,* 6(2): 175–200.

Williams, G. (1996a) Representing disability: some questions of phenomenology and politics, in C. Barnes and G. Mercer (eds) *Exploring the Divide: Illness and Disability.* Leeds: The Disability Press.

Williams, G. (1996b) Review essay: Irving Kenneth Zola (1935–1994), an appreciation, *Sociology of Health and Illness,* 18(1): 107–25.

Williams, R. (1979) *Politics and Letters.* London: Verso.

Williams, S. (1987) Goffman, interactionism, and the management of stigma in everyday life, in G. Scambler (ed.) *Sociological Theory and Medical Sociology.* London: Tavistock.

Williams, S. (1998) Capitalising on the emotions?, *Sociology,* 32(1): 121–39.

Wood, P. (1980) *International Classification of Impairments, Disabilities and Handicaps.* Geneva: World Health Organization.

Zarb, G. (1992) On the road to Damascus: first steps towards changing the relations of disability research production, *Disability, Handicap and Society,* 7(2): 125–38.

Zarb, G. (ed.) (1995) *Removing Disabling Barriers.* London: Policy Studies Institute.

Zarb, G. (1997) Researching disabling barriers, in C. Barnes and G. Mercer (eds) *Doing Disability Research.* Leeds: The Disability Press.

Zarb, G. and Oliver, M. (1992) *Ageing with a Disability: The Dimensions of Need.* London: Thames Polytechnic.

Zarb, G. and Nadash, P. (1994) *Cashing in on Independence.* Derby: BCODP.

Zola, I.K. (1982) *Ordinary Lives: Voices of Disease and Disability*. Watertown, MA: Apple-wood Books.

Zola, I.K. (1991) Bringing our bodies and ourselves back in: reflections on a past, present, and future 'medical sociology', *Journal of Health and Social Behaviour*, 32(March): 1–16.

Zola, I.K. (1993) Self, identity and the naming question: reflections on the language of disability, *Social Science and Medicine*, 36: 267–73.

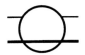

Index